ROUTLEDGE LIBRARY EDITIONS:
PUBLIC POLICY

Volume 2

FAMILY DOCTORS AND PUBLIC POLICY

FAMILY DOCTORS AND PUBLIC POLICY

A Study of Manpower Distribution

JOHN R. BUTLER

in collaboration with
J. M. BEVAN AND R. C. TAYLOR

Routledge
Taylor & Francis Group
LONDON AND NEW YORK

First published in 1973 by Routledge & Kegan Paul Ltd.

This edition first published in 2026
by Routledge
4 Park Square, Milton Park, Abingdon, Oxon OX14 4RN

and by Routledge
605 Third Avenue, New York, NY 10158

Routledge is an imprint of the Taylor & Francis Group, an informa business

British Library Cataloguing in Publication Data
A catalogue record for this book is available from the British Library

ISBN: 978-1-041-10085-0 (Set)
ISBN: 978-1-041-08914-8 (Volume 2) (hbk)
ISBN: 978-1-041-08926-1 (Volume 2) (pbk)
ISBN: 978-1-003-64757-7 (Volume 2) (ebk)

DOI: 10.4324/9781003647577

Family doctors and public policy

A study of manpower distribution

John R. Butler

Health Services Research Unit
University of Kent

in collaboration with

J. M. Bevan and R. C. Taylor

Routledge & Kegan Paul

London and Boston

First published in 1973
by Routledge & Kegan Paul Ltd
Broadway House, 68–74 Carter Lane,
London EC4V 5EL and
9 Park Street,
Boston, Mass. 02108, U.S.A.
Printed in Great Britain by
C. Tinling & Co. Ltd, London and Prescot

ISBN 0 7100 7640 1

Library of Congress Catalog Card No. 73-79109

Contents

Preface and acknowledgments

The research project out of which this book has grown originated in a research proposal submitted by two of us (JMB and RCT) to the Department of Health and Social Security in 1968. The research grant resulting from this submission enabled the third member (JRB) to join the team in 1969 and to assume primary responsibility for the fieldwork and for writing the report of the study. The full report, of which this book is an abbreviated version, was submitted to the DHSS on completion of the study in December 1971.

Many people have contributed in various ways to the research, and we gratefully acknowledge all their help, advice, assistance and encouragement. We are especially indebted to the following.

From the Department of Health and Social Security, Dr J. E. Struthers, Dr T. S. Eimerl, Mr F. W. Harris, Dr A. Bryce Stewart, Dr G. Sichel, Mr K. M. Francis, Mr J. Gallehawk, Mr C. J. Nickless, Mr D. A. Austin and Mr T. I. Butler.

The Divisional Medical Officers, Dr J. Mackellar, Dr E. D. Robb, Dr H. A. Tuck, Dr G. W. Whittall, Dr R. W. Bone and Dr A. W. Lilley, each of whom undertook a large amount of administrative work in connection with the survey.

The Regional Medical Officers, too numerous to mention individually, who kindly agreed to sign the original covering letter and deal with enquiries from doctors in their areas arising from the survey.

Dr A. Maiden and Mr L. Fisher of the Medical Practices Committee.

Dr D. L. Gullick and his colleagues at the British Medical Association.

Mr D. C. Bowie of the British Postgraduate Medical Federation.

The 1,721 general practitioners who took precious time at a peak workload period to complete the questionnaire. The cloak of anonymity precludes us from naming them individually, but to them we are especially grateful.

Our colleagues at the University of Kent, especially Miss

C. M. Marsh, Miss J. Dobby, Dr K. S. Dawes and Professor M. D. Warren.

The many secretaries, typists and willing helpers who have contributed much to the practical business of doing research and writing a book, Pat Bevan, Gill Butler (and the coding team), Denise Matthews, Angela Townsend, Kathleen Goldsmith, Jacquie Aldridge, Shirley Woodward and Lynn Browne.

We now realise why authors at this stage traditionally avow that, after receiving such expert help, any errors and omissions are their responsibility alone. We happily subscribe to the tradition.

John R. Butler, John M. Bevan
University of Kent

Rex Taylor
University of Aberdeen

Introduction

This is a study of inequalities in the distribution of general medical practitioners. It attempts to clarify the extent of the problem over time and space, to identify the underlying determinants and correlates, and to assess the effect of ameliorative measures. The study is limited to general practitioners in England: doctors working in hospitals or local authorities are excluded and so too (for reasons given later, p. 44) are GPs in Wales and Scotland. There is also a temporal limitation, for although it is broadly concerned with patterns of distribution throughout the lifetime of the National Health Service, the detailed research underlying the study is concerned mainly with the present situation. While these limitations were considered necessary in order to facilitate our contribution to future policy decisions, they do not exclude the possibility that this study might have wider interest and relevance. In this sense it is not only a detailed study of the unequal distribution of GPs in England but also a case-study in the unequal provision of social services.

This unequal provision has been of growing interest to social scientists in recent years, and a number of studies have documented the phenomenon in relation to a wide variety of services. Mention of just one or two such studies must suffice to familiarise the reader with the substantial disparities which have been found between areas. Cooper and Culyer's study of the fifteen hospital regions in England and Wales analysed regional inequalities in both the provision and the quality of services.[1] They utilised eleven separate indices of provision, including the number of hospital beds, the population per hospital doctor and consultant and *per capita* expenditure on hospitals. Overall, there was considerable regional variation, and regions which performed poorly on one index also performed poorly on the others. For example, the Oxford Region was better served than the Sheffield Region on all eleven indices. More important, those areas with a shortage of general practitioners also tended to have fewer hospital beds and doctors, a lower expenditure per in-patient week and a lower expenditure *per capita* at risk. Correspondingly, waiting lists and average hospital stay tended to be longer. Variation in the quality of services was studied obliquely through a regional analysis of Consultant Distinction Awards for the period 1960–6. Cooper and Culyer found that in each year, and for each of the four categories of award, the Oxford and Metropolitan Regions had the highest percentage of consultants receiving distinction awards, Wessex had the lowest, and there was relatively little stability of ranking among the rest. They acknowledge the difficulties in deriving objective statistical measures of quality, but are nevertheless forced to conclude that 'under the NHS as it currently is, the quality [of care] the average patient receives is determined chiefly by geography'.

The most comprehensive recent assessment of regional variation in local authority provision of health and welfare services is summarised in Appendix G of the Report of the Committee on Local Authority and Allied Personal Social Services.[2] Ranges of provision between 173 local health and welfare authorities are given for eleven different services in 1965, including special housing for the elderly, health visitors, home helps, mental health social workers and other social workers. The main results are summarised in Table 1. Clearly, the

Table 1 Regional variations in Local Authority provision of health and welfare services

	Average for England and Wales (per 1,000 population)	Number of authorities with less than the national average provision	Number of authorities with less than half the national average provision
Persons in special housing for the elderly	10·9	126	87
Health visitors	0·12	65	3
Home helps	0·63	97	7
Mental health workers	0·03	35	5
Home nurses	0·18	84	1
Other social workers	0·05	78	12

variations revealed in the provision of these six services do not require exhaustive supplementation to justify the conclusion of the Seebohm Committee that there are 'considerable differences in the quantity of services provided in different areas [and that this] unevenness does not bear any systematic relationship to differences in local need'.

Dental services are subject to similar regional variations. Studies by Walker *et al.*[3] and Cook and Walker[4] show a range in the ratio of dentists per 1,000 population from 0·09 in Hartlepool to 0·53 in Chester and Eastbourne. Of the ten executive councils with the best ratios of dentists per population, eight were located south of a line running from the Trent to the Severn, while seven of the worst ten executive councils in this respect were located north of this line. Generally, dentists in the north of England, the Midlands and Wales had twice as many potential patients as those working in the south-east. Not surprisingly, the main conclusion offered by Cook and Walker is that there is 'a gross regional imbalance' in the distribution of dentists.

Finally, Maynard's recent study provides evidence of significant variations between Regional Hospital Boards in both the provision and quality of psychiatric care in England and Wales.[5] In 1967 the range of provision was from 3·2 beds per 1,000 population in the Sheffield Region to 7·8 beds per 1,000 population in the South-West Metropolitan Region. The ratio for England and Wales was 4·2. Like Cooper and Culyer, Maynard is cautious about measuring variations in quality of service, but he uses the ratio of specialist staff per 100 hospital residents as a 'proxy of quality'. For consultants in psychiatry the regional range was from 0·44 in the South-West to 1·05 in the Oxford region; for psychologists, it was from 0·11 in the South-West to 0·58 in the North-West Metropolitan Region, and for social workers, from 0·25 in East Anglia to 0·76, again in the North-West Metropolitan Region. The ranges for instructors and nurses were of similar magnitude and tended to confirm the East Anglian and South-Western Regions as the least well-endowed and the Oxford and North-West Metropolitan as the best-endowed regions. Maynard therefore concluded 'that there are substantial inequalities and that there is no evidence to show that regions that are badly endowed in one sphere are compensated by better endowments in other spheres'.

Having placed the maldistribution of general practitioners in the context of regional variations in the provision of other health and welfare services, it is necessary to go one step further to provide a final and more general context for the present study. All public services, from housing through health and welfare to transport and recreation, have a latent redistributive function.[6] By adding in various ways to the total welfare of the individual, through the provision of goods and services financed by differential taxation, they redistribute some of the wealth from the relatively rich to the relatively poor. The greater the provision of public services, the greater the potential redistributive effect. Variations in either the provision or the consumption of public services generate inequalities of opportunity to make the most of life. Social scientists have tended to concentrate on variations in *consumption*, and they have shown for example that the use of most public educational, health and recreational services declines with social class.[7] This under-use of services weakens the redistributive effect and strengthens those inequalities resulting from *class* position. Such studies confirm the view that inequality follows a vertical distribution. By contrast, a study of variations in the *provision* of public services contributes to our understanding of inequalities resulting from *spatial* position. Here inequality follows a horizontal distribution. This form of inequality has always been implicit in the 'two nations' claim and in rural–urban comparisons, but it is only in the last decade that the concept of 'spatial inequality' has been used explicitly in relation to social and welfare services.[8] Local authorities differ not only in wealth but also 'in the rules they adopt for the allocation of public services and facilities; they differ in the number and degree of skills of the professional gatekeepers they employ; they differ in the system of administration and organisation which they adopt and the degree of cooperation and coordination which may exist between "chief officers" and the rest of their managerial staff'.[9]

The use of the concept 'spatial inequality' involves the suggestion that position in space – local authority, county, region – can operate independently of vertical or class position in determining life chances and life styles. A hypothetical example will make this clear. Consider two families with wage-earners in manual occupations. The first family lives in an economically prosperous region and in a local authority area with a good supply of houses, new schools, day nurseries and other social services. Bus services are frequent and there are a number of public parks. The family lives in a teaching hospital region and in an area with a good supply of dentists, doctors and social workers. The second family lives in an economically depressed region and in an area relatively poorly supplied in each of these amenities. To the extent that a relative abundance of such amenities and services endows people with a substantial headstart in life, it is clear that the first family in this example is more advantageously placed than the second, even though their positions in the social stratification system may be very similar. This family is in a better position to realise what Marshall calls 'the legitimate expectations of citizenship'.[10]

Since the introduction of a *National* Health Service in 1948, access to a general practitioner has been one of these legitimate expectations.

It is guaranteed by law. But some citizens have been less fortunate than others. The present study is concerned with the attempt to remedy this situation. The opening chapter makes it clear that the Ministry of Health inherited the problem in 1948, and, despite the use of both negative controls and positive incentives, has been unable to eliminate the unequal distribution. Attempts at redistribution during the first twenty years of the National Health Service were restricted principally to the powers of negative direction operated by the Medical Practices Committee. Following the Charter for the Family Doctor Service of 1965 and the Seventh Report of the Review Body on Doctors' and Dentists' Remuneration, issued in May 1966, these were supplemented by a positive incentive. The Review Body fixed the incentive payment at £400 per annum, payable to general practitioners practising in areas which had been continuously designated as short of doctors for a period of three years. This became known as the designated area allowance. Initially the profession reacted favourably, but increasingly throughout 1967 they advanced many detailed criticisms, and by 1968 they favoured a completely new scheme. At this juncture, in the summer of 1968, we were invited by the Department of Health to submit proposals for 'a short research project on the effectiveness of the incentive allowance in attracting GPs to Designated Areas'. The invitation was accepted on condition that the enquiry be extended to include, first, an analysis of the differences, real and apparent, between GPs work and living conditions in designated and non-designated areas, and second, a more general study of mobility and the factors affecting mobility among GPs. The scope of the research was later extended still further to include a detailed analysis of the regional pattern in the attraction and retention of family doctors.

The research was completed in 1971 and submitted to the Department of Health and Social Security as a Report on the Designated Area Study. The present work is a considerably shortened version of this Report. In presenting it now to a wider public we are conscious of widespread topical interest not only in the problem of under-doctored areas as such, but, since maldistribution is generic to the social services, in conceptual distinctions and methods of analysis as well. In particular, we hope that future discussions of maldistribution will be improved by our distinction between 'extensiveness' and 'intensiveness' and between problems of 'attraction' and 'retention', and that future researchers will find it useful to expand our analysis of mobility propensities and career patterns.

1 The history of the designated areas

Neither the BMA nor the Ministry have ever seriously thought about places which don't attract enough doctors. They can't have!

GP in Yorkshire

The background to the National Health Service Act

A major aim of the 1946 National Health Service Act was to achieve a fairer distribution of medical care resources than under the pre-war system. There is some disagreement about the real extent of maldistribution of doctors in the decade before the war, but most commentators agree not only that a wide gulf existed between areas with the best and worst provisions, but also that these differences corresponded roughly with the socio-economic composition of communities. Titmuss, for example, notes that 'the gross overcrowding of the London specialist population was accompanied by an abundance of general practitioners in the well-to-do and supposedly healthier districts',[1] and Eckstein records that 'places like Harrogate were gorged with general practitioners while working class areas nearby, in cities like Wakefield, Leeds and Bradford were comparatively starved for them'.[2] The PEP Broadsheet of 1944, from which both Titmuss and Eckstein drew much of their data, commented that the existing distribution of medical resources was 'at present haphazard ... and determined primarily by the income level or the rateable capacity of the locality. The National Health Insurance [NHI] scheme [dating from 1911] does not appear to have influenced the distribution of doctors in more than a minor degree ... and one of the 1944 White Paper's reasons for rejecting a mere extension of health insurance is that the NHI scheme affords no effective means of ensuring a proper distribution of doctors.'[3] In spite of a few cautionary opinions, notably from the Jewkeses,[4] who rightly draw attention to the inadequacies of evaluating distribution solely in terms of relative population sizes, it seems safe to conclude that the concern about uneven list sizes expressed from many quarters during the years leading up to the 1946 Act reflected a situation in which there was not only a substantial and indefensible geographical maldistribution of doctors, but also where the natural forces tending towards equalisation were at best very slight.[5]

The first mention of formal machinery to control the location of GPs seems to have been made in the 1944 White Paper[6] which envisaged the establishment of a central executive body, composed mainly of doctors and to be known as the Central Medical Board. The Board would, amongst other things, have powers of negative direction over GPs to influence their geographical distribution throughout the country. Following the publication of the White Paper a detailed questionnaire was sent to all members of the British Medical Association (BMA), the results of which showed a small majority of the medical profession as a whole (57 per cent) and also of general practitioners (51 per cent) to be in favour of the proposed measures, but the poll was repudiated by the Association's leaders.[7] In the ensuing discussions the profession's negotiators seem to have persuaded the government to drop the idea of control by the Central Medical Board, for no mention of it appeared in the revised plan.[8] Instead the Ministry proposed a part-salary element in the system of remuneration which could be varied to attract doctors to needy areas.[9] The satisfaction which the BMA leaders doubtless felt from their success in these negotiations was, however, short-lived. In the 1945 general election the Labour Party was returned to power not only committed in large measure to the 1944 White Paper, but also with a powerful and resolute Minister of Health in the person of Aneurin Bevan. When the National Health Service Bill was eventually published in 1946 it contained legislative proposals for a new central Medical Practices Committee (MPC), and it reverted to the earlier idea of the White Paper by giving the Committee powers of negative control over the residential settlement of GPs. The Bill, understandably, angered the BMA, and yet another plebiscite was organised; but the cause was hopeless and after an uneventful passage through Parliament the Bill became law in November 1946. Section 34 of the Act required the Minister to appoint a Medical Practices Committee, and thus was institutionalised the means of controlling the distribution of family doctors.

1948–61: post-war improvements

Right up to the appointed day in 1948 the BMA continued to resist any threat to the freedom of movement of doctors, and the Medical Practices Committee was constituted in an atmosphere of hostility and suspicion, even though seven of its nine members were doctors. But by the end of 1948 the Association had begun to temper its hostility in the light of the experience of GPs embarking upon National Health Service practice. As more people registered with their doctors before and after 5 July, the uneven distribution of practitioners became increasingly apparent. Some found they had very small lists of NHS patients, and within the first few months of the new service many were applying to the MPC to have their areas declared over-doctored and thus closed to new applicants.[10] Negative direction had begun, largely on the initiative of the rank-and-file members of the profession.

The early fears of the BMA about the role of the Medical Practices Committee were in fact to prove groundless. In its first report in June 1949 the Committee noted that the steady expansion in the number of doctors and the introduction of inducement payments had already begun to effect the redistribution of practitioners. Instead of taking drastic redeployment action the Committee therefore began to develop criteria for classifying medical practice areas, based upon data and recommendations from the local executive councils.[11] Four types of area were originally created, but, following the Danckwerts award in 1952 (one element of which was to discourage large list sizes), these were reduced to three. A fourth type was restored in 1962 and the current classification (1972) is shown in Table 2.

Table 2 The four types of practice area

Type of practice area	Average list size	Right to practise
Restricted	under 1,800	Normally refused
Intermediate	1,800–2,000	Problematic
Open	2,100–2,500	Automatic
Designated	over 2,500	Encouraged

In designated areas the right of practice was (and still is) automatically recognised, and doctors wishing to set up new practices in these areas were encouraged to do so through a financial grant known originally as the fixed annual payment and changed in 1952 to the initial practice allowance.[12] In open areas admission to the medical list is usually automatic; in intermediate areas applications might be refused; and in restricted areas applications are normally refused, even as replacements for outgoing practitioners.

The combination of negative direction and certain positive financial incentives worked well in the early years of the service while the number of incoming family doctors was increasing. Indeed, by 1951 the question was being raised of whether too many doctors were entering general practice. The evidence showed that a permanent position (i.e. as a principal or assistant with a view to partnership) was difficult to achieve, and a *Lancet* editorial in August of that year concluded that England and Wales had an annual surplus approaching 200 general practitioners.[13] However, the effect of the fierce competition for partnerships (there were as many as 100 applicants for each vacancy) hastened the movement of doctors to the most needy places, and the Medical Practices Committee was able to note in 1953 that there had been an 11 per cent increase in the number of doctors in areas which had been designated in 1948 and a decrease of almost 10 per cent in restricted and intermediate areas. The result was a rapid 'de-designation' of many areas, a trend which continued throughout the decade (see Appendix A, Table A1). The period between 1952 and 1961 unquestionably saw a dramatic reduction in the extensiveness of designated areas in England and Wales: the percentage of NHS patients in these places fell from 52 to a mere 17, and the number of principals fell from 7,596 in 1952 to 2,888 in 1961.

By the middle of the decade all the statistical indications seemed favourable, and hardly any public or professional concern was expressed over the distribution of GPs. Rather, the continuing unease within the profession centred around a potential overloading of the market. Even the Medical Practices Committee had raised the question in 1954 of whether an excess of general practitioners might not be in sight. In the same year the Cohen Committee[14] advocated an enquiry into the need for controlling the intake of medical students, and the new committee, chaired by Sir Henry Willinck, was constituted the following year. In its report in 1957 the majority of the committee proposed a 10 per cent decrease in the intake of medical students from the earliest possible date.[15] There appeared at the time to be many cogent reasons for accepting this recommendation, for all the evidence seemed to indicate a dwindling demand for medical manpower, but it soon became clear that the findings of the committee were based upon inaccurate population projections and forecasts.[16] In any case the intake of medical students had been declining in the years leading up to 1957, and the medical schools made no move to accelerate the rate of decrease.

1961–6: the formulation of a policy

For a few more years the proportions of principals and patients in designated areas continued to fall, but the effect of the reduced intake of medical students in the latter half of the 1950s began to appear in the early 1960s in the dwindling output of British graduates.[17] Only 1,511 British medical students graduated in 1963–4 at a time when more doctors were choosing hospital careers and many were emigrating.[18,19] Consequently the supply of general practitioners failed to keep pace with population growth, and from 1958 onwards the average list size of principals in England and Wales rose steadily (Table A1). By 1966 it had passed the high point of 1952, and by 1969 the average for the country as a whole was only twenty-one short of designation. The trend was also reflected in the spread of the designated areas: increasing numbers of areas were becoming designated as list sizes crept up everywhere. Between 1961 and 1970 the proportion of patients in these areas increased from 17 per cent to 36 per cent and of principals from 14 per cent to 32 per cent.

The medical profession's concern over this changing situation was first evident in 1961 when the General Medical Services Committee (GMSC) debated a motion that extra money should be used to attract more practitioners into the designated areas.[20] In fact the debate ended inconclusively, but it was important in being the first time since 1948 that the possibility was discussed in high circles of supplementing the negative control of the Medical Practices Committee with positive financial incentives. The theme was taken up again in 1963 by the Gillie Committee on the Field of Work of the Family Doctor, which noted that the post-war improvement in the distribution of GPs had apparently stopped and expressed the view that 'more should be done to distribute doctors more evenly throughout the country, not only by the work of the Medical Practices Committee, but by greater financial incentives to practise in under-doctored areas and by the provision of premises by local housing authorities in those areas'.[21] In the following year (1964) the Working Party on General Practice could not escape the conclusion 'that further redistribution is desirable, and that measures must be considered not only to increase the relative attractiveness of the under-doctored areas but also to restrict the further possibility of entry into practice in the most favoured areas'.[22] In the face of such mounting pressure the Medical Practices Committee informed the profession in June 1964 that it proposed to increase the number of restricted and intermediate areas, thereby diverting new applicants away from a greater number of desirable areas.[23]

This action was not at all to the profession's liking, and the GMSC vigorously reaffirmed its abhorrence of any form of direction and its belief in the selective use of positive financial incentives in areas with large lists and high morbidity rates.[24] By the end of that year (1964) the principle of financial inducements seems to have been widely accepted and the debate switched to the method of payment – whether it should be a lump sum or recurrent, and whether it should be paid from the pool.[25] The latter question was effectively resolved in the Charter for the Family Doctor Service, published in March 1965, which, by abolishing the pool entirely, heralded the most fundamental change in methods of remuneration and terms of service of general practitioners since the inception of the NHS.[26] But the Charter failed to give a clear lead on a policy for designated areas. In a remarkably vague paragraph dealing with the general problem of under-doctored areas (22b) the BMA simply stated: 'it is essential that the government should provide greater inducements in [these] special areas. We favour such a method rather than any form of direction.' Faced with such a general demand the Ministry could do no more than comment that 'the Association gives no indication of the form they consider the proposed inducements should take'.[27]

The local medical committees and the BMA promptly accepted the Ministry's offer to negotiate on the Charter, and agreed also that the new contract of service should be priced by the Review Body on Doctors' and Dentists' Remuneration. The interim reports of the negotiations which followed indicated that both sides were aware of the complexity of the problem of under-doctored areas and were anxious to consider the broadest possible range of solutions. In their first report, for example, the negotiators expressed concern that doctors in these areas should look forward not simply to proper financial rewards but to 'conditions of work which are professionally satisfying both in their own practices and in their relationships with other services'.[28] But, for whatever reasons, these ideals were eventually abandoned in favour of the cruder (but presumably more feasible) solution of money. The second report of the joint discussions, in October 1965, contained the crucial paragraph which was eventually to form the basis for the new deal.[29] 'The basic practice allowance for doctors in areas where there is a long-standing shortage of GPs will be increased. This will include all doctors whose main surgery is situated in the defined area, and all patients on such a doctor's list will be counted in determining eligibility. The appropriate areas will be those which have been "designated" by the Medical Practices Committee for a continuous period of three years up to the date of payment. This criterion will be kept under review.'

Following the negotiations between the BMA and the Ministry the new contract was priced by the Review Body in its much-heralded seventh report in May 1966.[30] The additional allowance for practice in designated areas was covered in paragraph 206. The Review Body considered the allowance to be a straight inducement payment which, by virtue of its novelty, could not be fixed precisely. The report acknowledged ignorance of what figure would constitute a realistic inducement, or even of how far a reluctance to practise in these areas could be overcome by financial payments; but members were concerned that the amount should be sufficiently low to prevent a catastrophic loss of earnings when an area ceased to be designated. The figure eventually decided was £400 per annum, payable when an area had been continuously designated by the MPC for a period of three years.

1966–9: dissatisfaction with the designated area allowance

The BMA's reaction to the Review Body report was mostly favourable, although the new allowance was less well received. In the course of a number of meetings of various committees during the summer of 1966 many detailed criticisms were levelled against the new allowance: that payment should not be tied absolutely to a three-year qualifying period; that GPs in under-doctored areas might not want to improve the position since it would hasten the loss of their allowance; that doctors would not be attracted by £400 because areas might well lose their designation as soon as they arrived; and that the criteria for designation should extend beyond that of doctor/patient ratios to include the existence of social and cultural activities, educational facilities, physical characteristics, population density, morbidity patterns, the incidence of chronic occupational disease, and the adequacy of supporting medical services.[31] This latter argument was taken up again by the General Medical Services Committee at meetings early in 1967 when the Committee was considering a complaint from the Glamorgan local medical committee that whilst the Rhondda Valley was not a designated area, Abingdon in Berkshire *was* designated.[32,33] The Welsh representatives argued that such factors as morbidity, educational and cultural facilities, and the number of items of service rendered per £1,000 paid should be taken into account in deciding whether or not an area should be designated. A large list size, they told the Committee, was the least difficulty in filling vacancies in the Rhondda: the real deterrents included excessive workloads, high morbidity, the forbidding nature of the Welsh mining valleys, difficulties in obtaining building sites, and the absence of cultural and other amenities. The long-term solution should be for medical assessors to visit such areas and assess their true circumstances and needs in depth.

These arguments, which appeared again at the British Medical Association's annual representative meeting in 1967,[34] appear to confuse two separate issues. There is much force in the argument that list size is a poor indicator of the demand for primary medical care and hence of the need for manpower. It is true that, all else being equal, the workload on each doctor is likely to be greater in areas with high lists than in those with lower average lists, but in practice all else is not equal, and a simple relationship between list size and workload does not always hold good. Many factors in addition to list size affect the pattern of utilisation of services and standards of care, and these should ideally be taken into account in deciding whether or not more practitioners are needed. That argument has much to commend it, but to link it with the argument about social and environmental considerations is to confuse the issue, for the payment of extra money to doctors in areas which are socially or culturally unattractive, *regardless* of their medical needs or whether they are under-doctored, would be akin to a straight compensation payment of a kind that was not intended by the Review Body at all, and that would not necessarily improve the distribution of manpower on any relevant criteria.

Whatever the intrinsic merits of these arguments, they appear to have swayed the Minister, who acknowledged in June 1967 that the problems of chronically designated areas could not adequately be met merely by additional payments; but he did no more than introduce a number of small administrative changes in the regulations governing payment of the allowance.[35] He may have been hoping that the whole question would be re-examined by the Review Body, and it was with this end in view also that the BMA submitted a further memorandum of evidence, in October, which again reflected the profession's desire to devise a radically new system.[36] In this memorandum the Association pointed out that the designated area allowance was not having the intended effect and that discussions with the Ministry had not substantially changed the criteria for payment. Two interim measures were proposed for the Review Body's consideration pending a full review of the entire scheme: first, that the allowance should be increased and paid over a much longer period; and second, that the rules governing the de-designation of areas should be liberalised to reduce the impact of losing the allowance.

When the Review Body did eventually pronounce, in its ninth report in May 1968, it disappointed many expectations.[37] The report re-emphasised the experimental nature of the scheme and re-stated the case for keeping the level of payment low, but it did not alter the amount of the allowance or the rules governing its payment. In fact the only concessions made with respect to under-doctored areas were that the three-year period of qualification should be kept under continuous review, and that the Health Departments and the profession's representatives might take a joint initiative in making arrangements for an increase in the allowance and in submitting any such proposals to the Review Body. It seems, however, that the members were thinking in terms of fairly small increases, for they specifically commented that 'there would be no difficulty in justifying an increase of, say, £100 under the "manpower" criterion of current incomes policy'. The reaction of the profession was, expectedly, swift and derogatory. At a special conference of representatives of local medical committees in June 1968 the motion was carried that 'this conference is of the opinion that following receipt of the Review Body's report, under-doctored areas can only look forward to a further deterioration in manpower, and that further additional payments should be sought to attract practitioners to these areas. This should be a realistic inducement to the order of, say, £1,000 per annum. . . .'[38] The debate was fierce and bitter, but even by then negotiations were under way with the Ministry on the whole future of the scheme.

1969–72: the search for improvements

The outcome of the negotiations was known in July 1969 when the Health Departments made new proposals for a two-level system of payments to replace the existing flat-rate allowance.[39] It was suggested that the current allowance of £400 should continue to be paid to doctors in designated areas for as long as they remained in the same practice, or until they became entitled to a higher allowance of £500 payable to practitioners in designated areas with average lists in excess of 3,000. The higher rate would be paid when areas had been continuously designated for two years (as opposed to three years for the lower rate), and would continue for a further two years after de-designation. In considering these proposals the General Medical Services Committee again attacked the whole principle of designation and stressed the desirability of channelling extra resources into areas where workloads and morbidity rates were high rather than areas which simply had large average lists. One member even suggested that the profession's responsibility lay more in making the public aware of deficiencies in the service than in helping the government with short-sighted plans for relieving the under-doctored areas. But once again the Committee was unable to resolve the conflict between what ideally needed to be done and what was feasible and realistic with existing resources of manpower, money, knowledge and techniques. In the end, therefore, the Committee endorsed the principle of a two-level system of payments, adding additional recommendations that would give doctors in the designated areas even more money.

Eventually a 'limited agreement' was reached between the Health Departments and the profession's representatives, and the proposal was put to the Review Body in October 1969 that the designated area allowance should be paid in two amounts.[40,41] The first, for GPs in designated areas with average lists of between 2,500 and 2,999, would be payable after the area had been designated for three years and would continue for three years after de-designation. The higher allowance would be payable in areas which had been continuously designated for one year with average lists of 3,000 or more, and would continue for two years after the list size fell below this figure, when the lower rate would then be paid in the normal way. There was, however, no agreement between the two sides on the actual size of the allowances. The BMA argued that they should be of the order of £500 and £700 if they were to continue to act as material inducements. The Health Departments, on the other hand, took the view that the allowance had already proved effective and that the need for more doctors in areas where average lists were only a little above 2,500 was less than it had been. They also pointed out the need to prevent a sudden migration of GPs from areas which, though not actually designated, were nevertheless far from being over-doctored; and stressed the undesirability of large reductions in income for practitioners who ceased to be eligible. In the light of all these considerations the Departments recommended £400 and £550 as appropriate amounts.

The twelfth report of the Review Body, in June 1970, caused an immediate furore.[42] The report recommended across-the-board increases of 30 per cent for the whole of the medical profession, but the government agreed to pay the full amount only to the training grades, and in the case of other grades to pay half the increase immediately and to refer the remainder to the National Board for Prices and Incomes. The members of the Review Body instantly resigned *en bloc*. The anger of the BMA exceeded even that of the earlier comparable situation in 1966.[43] But the focus of the storm, as the BMA leaders repeatedly stressed, was on the principle of the government's action rather than any substantive contents of the report. This is, for our purposes, a matter of regret, for there is little evidence of the profession's reaction to the substantial increases proposed in the designated area allowance. The Review Body accepted the principle of a two-level system of payment, but the members must have concluded that even the BMA had under-stated its case, for they finally recommended that 'the upper level of the allowance be fixed at £849 and that the lower level should be increased to £519'. The report argued that the upper level was justified by the very high lists in some areas ('where average lists are 3,000 or more, the average is as high as 3,500'), and the old argument that too high a level would cause substantial losses when it ceased to be payable was rebutted on the curious grounds that, as the prospect of de-designation in such areas was remote, 'we need not be seriously concerned about the financial consequences of such withdrawal . . . for the doctors involved'.

Events moved swiftly following publication of the report. The remuneration of doctors became an issue in the general election campaign currently under way, and in the election itself a new government was returned to power. In July 1970 the new Secretary of State for Social Services (Sir Keith Joseph) informed the BMA that, in return for full co-operation by doctors in fulfilling their NHS contracts, the government would withdraw the reference to the Prices and Incomes Board.[44] However, for 'compelling reasons' only a further 5 per cent increase would be paid to general practitioners (giving them 20 per cent in all), and would stand for one year only. Under the new regulations, a Type 1 allowance of £490 was paid from 1 April 1970 under the same conditions as had governed payment of the old allowance; and in addition a new Type 2 allowance of £750 was paid to practitioners whose surgeries were in areas continuously designated for *one* year with average lists of 3,000 or more. The closing scenes of the battle of the twelfth Review Body Report came early in September 1970, when it was reported to a meeting of Council of the BMA that 'both the Central Committee for Hospital Medical

Services and the General Medical Services Committee had authorised their representatives to agree to the appropriate increase in salary scales and fees and allowances consequent on the government's decision on the twelfth report'.[45]

Thus for a while the storm has abated. A new Review Body was constituted in July 1971 under the chairmanship of Lord Halsbury and reported with remarkable speed in December that year.[46] Broadly speaking, the new Review Body restored the cuts made by the previous government eighteen months earlier, but not wholly in the manner recommended in the twelfth report. Thus although general practitioners received an overall increase of 8 per cent this was achieved through additions to the basic and supplementary practice allowances, the capitation fees and certain other fees and expenses. The designated area allowances remained untouched. The reason for this, as the Review Body itself explained, was the need for a rapid review for 1971–2 pending a more comprehensive assessment later. In making such an assessment the members expressed their intention not to limit themselves exclusively to periodic evidence submitted to them by the government and the medical and dental associations, but to take account also of relevant research data from universities and similar institutions as well as the views and comments of a wide range of professional groups, government departments and industries. Among the relevant research data which the Review Body received early in 1972 was a copy of the report of this study, and when the second Halsbury report appeared in June 1972 the designated area allowance was the only one of the thirty-three items of fees and allowances which make up a GPs remuneration to remain unaltered.[47] All the other items rose, by amounts ranging from 3 to 254 per cent. The Review Body commented, with respect to the designated area allowance: 'A recent [and as yet unpublished] study by the Health Services Research Unit of the University of Kent has revealed grounds for doubt as to whether the payments in their present form are making an effective contribution towards solving the problem of under-doctored areas, and the matter is to be discussed between the Health Departments and the profession in the near future. In these circumstances we do not recommend any change in the amount of these payments at present . . .' It is with the study to which the Review Body referred that the remainder of this book is concerned.

2 Controls and incentives[1]

> £400 wouldn't lure me to Gateshead. By the time they've knocked off 8/3d. in the pound, what's left isn't worth two hoots.
>
> GP in Derbyshire

Changes in the total number of family doctors in the country as a whole, and in any particular locality, may result from one possible movement or a combination of possible movements. Gross gains to the stock of principals may be made from various sources including the following: (1) established doctors in other branches of the profession, such as hospital medicine, administration or public health; (2) younger doctors who are either preparing for a career in general practice or who must shortly make a career decision; (3) doctors practising or being trained in other countries; and (4) assistants in general practice who aspire to principal status. In addition, gross gains in any particular locality of the country may result from the internal migration of GPs, but in these cases the gains in one locality are inevitably offset by corresponding losses in another. Depletions to the stock of principals may occur through losses to (1), (3) and, exceptionally, (4) above, and also through deaths and retirements. Schematically these movements can be represented as in Diagram 1.

The net result of all these gains and losses over time will determine the magnitude of changes in the total number of GPs in the country as a whole, and also in whichever sub-areas one may be interested in. It follows, therefore, that the failure of any particular area (for example a medical practice area) to achieve or maintain a specified number of principals may be the outcome of one circumstance or a combination of circumstances. These circumstances, moreover, may vary from area to area. In one place the shortage of manpower may be attributable mainly to failure in recruiting younger doctors entering general practice for the first time; in another place it may result primarily from abnormally high losses of established GPs to other parts of the country. It also follows that an adequate solution to the maldistribution of practitioners would first require an accurate

GROSS GAINS FROM

other branches of the medical profession
junior/student doctors
doctors in other countries
assistants in general practice

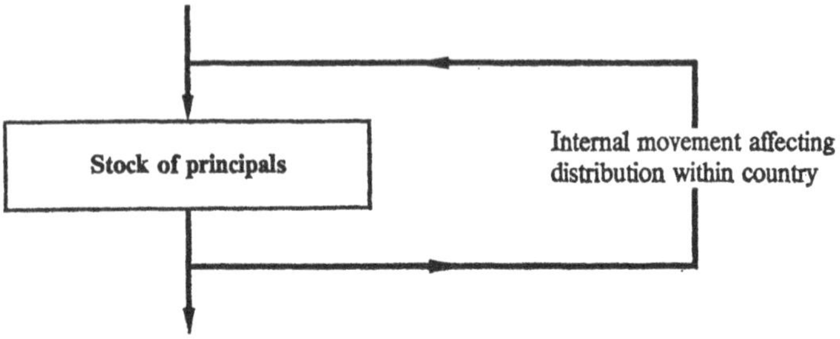

GROSS LOSSES TO

other branches of the medical profession
other countries
deaths and retirements

Diagram 1

diagnosis of the main reasons underlying the manpower shortage in different localities, and then a selective control over those processes which were shown to contribute most to the problem. In theory different policies may then be needed in different places, although it must obviously be acknowledged that in practice severe restraints exist upon the implementation of ideal policies.

However, before considering the feasibility of different policies (which is the concern of the concluding chapter) there must first be a logical analysis of the nature and causes of the problem, and an assessment of the value of existing policies. This chapter starts the analysis by outlining the mechanisms of intervention which are currently available to stimulate the supply of, and control the losses of, GPs at the local level. Then we consider possible criteria which might be used in assessing the effectiveness of these mechanisms; finally we apply these criteria in examining trends in the distribution of family doctors during the last twenty years.

Mechanisms of intervention

The entry of doctors into general practice is controlled statutorily by the local executive councils and the Medical Practices Committee, and may take one of several forms. When a doctor dies or resigns the executive council must immediately report to the MPC on the need for filling the vacancy. The council may consider that a successor is not needed and the report may recommend that the practice should be dispersed (in the case of a single-handed practice) or that the remaining partners should succeed to it (in the case of partnerships). If, however, the council feels that the vacancy should be filled, then a successor is appointed either by the existing partners or, in the case of a single-handed practice, by the Medical Practices Committee after consulting with the executive council and the local medical committee. The MPC retains control over the admission of new partners in restricted and intermediate areas, but provided the proposed partner is fully registered the Committee would never influence existing partners in their choice of a new colleague.

Another type of entry into general practice is created when an executive council, in consultation with the local medical committee, considers that a further doctor is needed in its area. The procedure for giving public notice of the vacancy and for selecting the candidates is the same as for the replacement of single-handed practitioners, with the MPC making the final selection. In addition, any doctor may himself apply for admission to the medical list of an executive council, and in such cases the council, again in consultation with the local medical committee, will consider the application and recommend to the MPC whether or not it should be allowed. The MPC is not bound to accept the council's recommendation, but the only statutory ground for refusal is that the area is already classified as restricted or intermediate.

A third route into general practice is via an assistantship. No direct control is exerted by the Medical Practices Committee in these cases, for a principal who wishes to employ an assistant for more than three months merely requires the approval of his executive council.[2] He may subsequently appeal to the MPC if his request is refused, but this appeals procedure is rarely used.[3] The salaries of assistants are paid directly by the principals who employ them, and an allowance of £700 (or £980 if it is accompanied by a designated area allowance) is made to principals employing full-time assistants. Relatively few doctors are now prepared to accept assistantships because of the ease with which ordinary and salaried partnerships can usually be obtained, and few of those who do accept such posts remain in them for long, but there may nevertheless be an important link between the distribution of assistants and the ultimate distribution of principals entering the medical list. Most assistants are young, with a considerable potential for geographical mobility, and if they can be encouraged to take assistantships in the less-well-doctored areas the prospects seem good of their becoming principals in those same areas.

Turning from the controls to the incentives, the most important inducement to stimulate GPs into moving to particular localities is the designated area allowance. This allowance, as noted in Chapter 1, developed out of the Family Doctor Charter in 1965, was priced at £400 by the Review Body in May 1966, and was first paid from 1 October that year, albeit at a reduced rate of £200 for the first six months. In April 1970 the new graduated payments of £490 and £750 were introduced. A doctor qualifies if he is eligible for the basic practice allowance and practises from a main surgery in an area that has been continuously designated by the Medical Practices Committee for at least three years (or one year in the case of the higher – Type 2 – allowance). The payment continues for a concessionary period of three years after the area ceases to be designated, or for two years in the case of the Type 2 allowance, after which doctors may continue to be eligible for the lower rate. As a result of these rather complex conditions of payment it is possible for GPs in some designated areas to be ineligible for the allowance (i.e. during the qualifying period), and, conversely, for doctors in some non-designated areas to be in receipt of it (i.e. during the concessionary period following de-designation). These anomalies, to which we return later, are important in assessing the effect of the allowance, for it can so far have had only a slight effect upon areas which did not immediately qualify, and virtually none upon those which had only just qualified three years after its introduction.

A medical practice area, which may vary in size from an entire county borough to a small section of a rural district, and whose boundaries may not coincide with those of any other administrative unit, is normally designated when the overspill of patients above an average of 2,500 per doctor exceeds 2,500 (which is the point at which one incoming doctor could set up a viable new practice). The deliberations of the Medical Practices Committee over the classification of areas are secret, but the impression is gained from official reports that the statistical criterion is fairly rigidly observed. Other relevant factors about an area in addition to average list size may be taken into account when the classification is borderline, but it seems as a rule that the Committee in England and Wales is somewhat less inclined than its Scottish counterpart to take account of the total situation. In deciding whether or not to designate a district, the Scottish MPC (an entirely separate body) considers many factors which vary from district to district, including the number of maternity cases dealt with, the number of temporary residents treated, the size of partnerships, and the amount of time spent on work other than general practice.[4] There is no rigid formula, and each case is considered on its merits.[5]

In addition to the designated area allowance, a further financial inducement exists for doctors to set up practice in these places – the initial practice allowance (IPA), payable whether or not the area also attracts the designated area allowance. Four types of initial practice allowance are paid depending upon the nature of the practice and the list size in the area. The basic purpose of the allowance is to provide an income 'cushion' for a period of between two and four years for GPs establishing themselves in a designated area, but although the amount of the allowance varies in a complex way from type to type, three of the four types are based upon a 'reckonable income' of at most £4,000 per annum. The number of doctors in England and Wales in receipt of an initial practice allowance is small (193 in 1970), and the total cost in 1970–1 was only £274,000 – little more than one-tenth of the cost of the designated area allowances.[6] The probable effect of the IPA on the overall distribution of practitioners is consequently quite small, although a survey conducted by the Health Departments in 1968 indicated that the Type A allowance (which is of much longer standing than the others) had been effective in establishing a number of doctors in single-handed practice in the designated areas.[7]

Criteria for assessing the effectiveness of the mechanisms of intervention

Before examining the impact of these controls and incentives upon the geographical distribution of family doctors, some attention must be paid to two methodological problems involved in making such an assessment. The first is the familiar problem in the social sciences of identifying the specific causes of change. Even if it could be shown that area inequalities had declined since 1948 it would not necessarily follow that this was due to the various administrative procedures described in the previous section. There is nothing in the nature of a control group to which we can turn for comparison, and we do not therefore know what would have happened if the old system had continued. People move more frequently now than thirty or forty years ago, and it is arguable that some spontaneous improvement might have occurred even if nothing had been done. There is no foolproof solution to the problem, but by a combination of the careful analysis of available evidence and common-sense judgments on matters where information is lacking, it is possible to form some impression of how well the mechanisms have been working. If, for example, there is evidence in the data of a long-term trend towards the equalisation of list sizes in different parts of the country, then we need not reject the proposition that some forms of intervention are at least doing no harm and may actually be contributing to the trends. Or again, if some significant changes are observed following the introduction or modification of a particular administrative measure (such as the designated area allowance) we could conclude that the measure had probably been a factor in bringing about the changes, especially if there is no evidence of any other variables which might reasonably be expected to produce a similar change. Again, however, it must be acknowledged that this could never be proven in any rigorous way because of the lack of a control group.

The second problem is rather more complex, and concerns the information that is accepted as valid evidence of a trend towards a fairer distribution of family doctors. The nub of the problem can be seen in considering the possible answers to the question: what is a fair distribution? It is clear that at least two different answers can be given, accepting for the time being that list size is the most practicable indicator of the need for manpower. One answer would describe a fair distribution as one in which as few patients as possible are on larger lists than the conventionally accepted maximum size for any one doctor. Since this maximum is currently about 2,500 (at least in terms of official policy), those who accept this definition of a 'fair distribution' would seek evidence of a desirable trend in the distribution of GPs in a decline in the number of designated areas and in the proportions of doctors and patients in them. But there is another possible answer to the question, namely that a fair distribution is one in which the *range* in list sizes between areas is as narrow as possible, thus ensuring that patients in different parts of the country have more or less equal access to the services of a family doctor. Using this definition, signs of an improvement in the distribution of GPs would be sought in a reduction in the range of list sizes between the best and the worst areas: this might, for example, be evidenced in a declining disparity over time between average list sizes in designated and restricted areas.

These two alternative definitions of a 'fair distribution' are mutually incompatible when the national average list size *exceeds* the conventionally agreed maximum for each doctor. In this case each concept of a fair distribution can be fully achieved only at the expense of the other. A simple hypothetical example will illustrate the point. Among a patient population of 49 million, served by 19,000 doctors, the mean list size would be 2,579. In achieving the first aim (that of securing the greatest possible number of patients on lists below 2,500) it would theoretically be possible to arrange the doctors and patients spatially in such a way that 95 per cent of the population were on average lists of 2,475. This, however, would leave the remaining 5 per cent of the population on average lists of 12,760 – a gross inequality in the light of the second concept of fairness. Alternatively, a distribution could theoretically be arranged whereby each doctor had exactly 2,579 patients on his list. This would be a perfect situation in terms of the second concept of fairness (since there would be no variation at all between different parts of the country), but it would mean that every single patient was on a list above 2,500.

When the national average list is *less than* the generally accepted maximum, then both definitions of fairness can be satisfied at once. This would have been the case in England in 1971 if the average list size for the whole country (2,460) had also been repeated evenly throughout all the medical practice areas. It is, however, quite impossible to envisage anything even approaching such a perfect distribution occurring spontaneously in a free society, and so in practice a judgment may have to be made on the value of a *tendency* to move towards one or the other objective. For example, at a time when the national average list size is *rising*, a reduction in the number of designated areas (a desirable goal relative to the first aim) will usually be achieved only at the expense of an increasing disparity between list sizes in the remaining designated areas and the rest of the country (an undesirable outcome relative to the second aim). A judgment must then be made about the relative values of the two objectives.

The interest in relating resources to population in this way is not merely academic, for different interpretations of a fair distribution may lead to very different conclusions about what is actually happening. The BMA, for example, has consistently interpreted an increasing number of patients in designated areas as evidence of the failure of the allowance, but in fact it is evidence of failure only in the context of the first concept of fairness which, as we have seen, may not be the best definition at a time when list sizes are increasing across the country. The Review Body, on the other hand, was clearly concerned in its twelfth report (in June 1970) with the problem of the range between list sizes, for the introduction of the two-level system of payment makes sense only in terms of this particular definition of the problem. Yet the effect of reducing the number of areas with very large lists would be to increase the overall number of designated and open areas unless the total stock of general practitioners could be simultaneously augmented. Here, then, lies the choice. Of the two extreme situations in the hypothetical example above it would presumably be preferable for all patients to be on lists of 2,579 (in effect, for all areas to be designated) than for 95 per cent to be on average lists of 2,475 and the remaining 5 per cent on lists of 12,760. These are the extreme cases, but they show that an increase in the number of patients in designated areas is not necessarily evidence of a worsening *distribution* of available manpower, even though it may well be a sign that more doctors are needed in total.

Trends in the distribution of family doctors

The arrangement of material in this section follows the distinction drawn above between different ways of evaluating the distribution of GPs. Starting with the first concept of a fair distribution, which in the context of this research is equated with a decline in the extensiveness of the designated areas throughout the country, the evidence in Table A1 showed that for ten years from 1952 onwards the percentage of principals in designated areas in England and Wales fell steadily. A similar trend occurred among the patient population, although these figures are not given in the table. 1962, however, represented the turning point, and from then onwards the numbers of doctors and patients in designated areas increased rapidly until by 1968 there were proportionately more than in any year since 1952. The introduction of the designated area allowance in 1966 had no immediate effect upon the trend, for between 1966 and 1968 the number of principals in these areas increased by almost 1,500 and of patients by nearly four million. There are, however, signs within the last two years that the trend may have been halted if not actually reversed, for between 1968 and 1970 the numbers and proportions of principals and patients in the designated areas actually fell for the first time in eight years.

The same conclusion can be drawn from a simple count of the

number of designated areas. In spite of the general policy of amalgamating smaller practice areas into larger units, the number of designated areas increased from 241 in 1966 to 323 in 1970, a rise from 14 per cent to 20 per cent of the total number of medical practice areas. Within the last year, however, there has been a slight drop in the number of these areas, although they still account for almost a fifth of all practice areas.

The steady accumulation of designated areas during the last few years has meant that areas which were designated when the allowance started in 1966 have generally remained designated, with an increasing proportion becoming eligible for payment of the allowance. Of the 242 designated areas at the start of the scheme which could still be traced in 1970, a total of 193 (80 per cent) remained designated; 45 (19 per cent) had become open areas; three were classified as intermediate, and one as restricted. A higher proportion of areas qualifying for immediate payment of the allowance in 1966 had remained designated than of those not qualifying (88 per cent against 74 per cent), but this does not necessarily reflect badly upon the allowance itself. It is probable that areas which were immediately eligible in 1966 (that is, those which had already been designated for three years) presented more chronic and intransigent problems than the remainder, and would therefore not be expected to show the same degree of improvement in subsequent years. Whether or not even the 12 per cent of these areas which later became de-designated would have done so in the absence of the allowance is a point for speculation. What does seem to be beyond doubt, however, is that the allowance has so far had little apparent success in diminishing the extensiveness of the designated areas.

It may, nevertheless, remain possible for an effective degree of redistribution to have taken place if there is evidence of a trend towards the equalisation of list sizes between areas. It may be held, in other words, that data concerning the *extent* of the problem is less appropriate at a time when list sizes everywhere are creeping up than evidence about the relative *depth* of deprivation in different localities. Where more and more patients and doctors each year are finding themselves in designated areas it would nevertheless be an indication of some form of positive redistribution that the gap between the best and the worst areas was narrowing.

The general movement in list sizes was discussed in Chapter 1, and the full figures are set out in Table A1. In England and Wales as a whole the average number of patients per principal decreased until

1958 and thereafter it rose until 1970. In the designated areas, by contrast, average lists have actually fallen each year since 1966. At a time when the designated areas were increasing numerically (1966–8) this fall in the average list size may be no more than an indication that average lists in the newly designated areas were quite close to 2,500. However, the continuing fall in average list sizes after 1968, when the rise in the number of designated areas at first slowed and then reversed, can, in conjunction with the opposite trend in the restricted areas, be taken as valid evidence of movement towards a more equal distribution of available manpower.

An alternative way of plotting the trend towards the equalisation of list sizes is by expressing the average list size in each type of practice area as a ratio of the national average. From about 1953–4 onwards these ratios remained more or less constant for a period of seven or eight years, even though the proportions of doctors and patients in the designated areas were steadily falling throughout this time. Although the extent of the problem was gradually shrinking, the difficulty of large lists in those areas which remained designated was not disproportionately eased. In recent years, however, there has been a slight reduction in the range of ratios between the designated and restricted areas. Between 1964 and 1970 the ratio in designated areas fell from 117 to 113 (England and Wales = 100), with a corresponding increase in the ratio for restricted areas from 74 to 77. These figures suggest that a gradual movement towards the equalisation of list sizes has been under way at least since 1964 (and probably since 1961, although the changed definition of restricted areas in 1964 obscures the situation). In 1964, for instance, the average list size in designated areas was 58 per cent greater than in the restricted areas, but by 1970 the excess had fallen to 48 per cent. This trend, which has intensified in the last three years, has now continued for long enough to encourage the hope that it may be more than a short-lived phenomenon.

A broad summary of the data presented in this section would divide the post-war period into the years before and after about 1961. Up to this date there was a substantial and regular improvement in the extent of the problem of designated areas: the number of such areas declined and so too did the proportions of doctors and patients in them. But list sizes in those places which did remain designated stayed as high as ever, in just the same way as those in the restricted areas stayed as low as ever. Since about 1961 the patterns have reversed: there has been a steady growth in the extent of the designated areas throughout the country, but at the same time also a gradual narrowing in the range of list sizes between the best- and the worst-endowed places. Only the most recent changes in the last year or two could be attributed to the introduction of the designated area allowance, and even then there can be no certainty that the small improvements noted in 1969 and 1970 were due to the effects of the allowance or to the net increase in the number of GPs in those years. It would be consistent with the data, and defensible on logical grounds, to argue that the growth and decline in the designated areas merely reflects, after an appropriate time lapse, the gains or losses to the total stock of GPs in the country. It may, in any case, still be too early to make a realistic assessment of the impact of the allowance. Quite apart from the fact that a widespread movement of doctors cannot be expected overnight under any circumstances, there remains the anomaly that by no means all the designated areas actually qualify for the allowance. It is estimated that only a little over half (55 per cent) of all the designated areas in 1970 were eligible, and whilst the proportion has been rising each year since 1966 it nevertheless means that for a large number of designated areas the allowance has not yet had time to act as an effective inducement.

Entrance into general practice

We conclude this chapter with a brief consideration of how effectively the Medical Practices Committee is fulfilling its responsibilities of negative control. Since all the deliberations of the Committee are secret there can be no certain knowledge of the basis on which decisions are made regarding the admission of individual practitioners into particular areas, but some tentative conclusions may reasonably be drawn from published information about the outcome of those decisions. A glance at the number of principals admitted to the Medical List each year might suggest that the whole problem could be solved by somehow channelling all of one year's intake into the designated areas. For instance, during the year ending 30 September 1968 (the latest year for which figures are available in this form) 1,062 principals were admitted to the List in England and Wales,[8] almost twice the number needed at that time to bring the average list size in each executive council down to 2,500. Of these admissions, however, 403 were to designated areas, almost all as replacements for outgoing practitioners,[9] and these doctors cannot therefore be included as part of the potential 'pool'. A further 458 admissions were to open areas, most of them also as replacements, and on the assumption that a failure to replace GPs in open areas would have resulted in their becoming designated, thereby defeating the object of the exercise, these too must be excluded. There remained, therefore, at most 201 extra doctors available to bolster the supply of practitioners in the designated areas – that is, all those who were in fact admitted to intermediate and restricted areas. The MPC's control over admissions to these areas may have meant that each one of the 201 cases was justified on its merits, yet it is worth noting that if the Committee had refused to accept any *replacements* in these areas the effect would have been to redistribute anything up to 200 doctors from these areas to those which were designated or open. (The precise figure is obviously unknowable because it depends upon the number of doctors who would have opted out of general practice entirely rather than accept a vacancy in an unfavoured locality.) The failure to replace doctors in restricted and intermediate areas must result in an increase in the average list sizes there, but this is an inevitable consequence of a successful redistribution, however it is achieved. There at least appears to be a case for the MPC to review its methods of procedure in such situations.

The situation of assistants is rather different, for the Medical Practices Committee has no jurisdiction over their employment. Nevertheless the geographical distribution of assistants has a two-fold significance. In the short term, assistants provide an extra pair of hands and ease the workload of principals. In the longer term, assistants become principals themselves in a fairly short time and, as we have suggested, the more assistants that can be employed in the chronically under-doctored areas the more are likely to become principals there. On both counts the geographical distribution of assistants is seriously discrepant with an optimum distribution. In general, regions and counties with the greatest shortages of family doctors (particularly the East and West Midlands and the Northern region) have the fewest assistants, whilst regions with the most assistants (notably the South-East) are relatively well supplied with principals.[10] As with admissions to the Medical List, there is no certain knowledge of the general grounds on which executive councils decide either to accept or reject an application to employ an assistant. It is not even known whether any serious attempt is made to control the number of assistants going into restricted or intermediate areas. In the absence of such knowledge it would be unwise to place too much emphasis on the possible benefits resulting from an extension of the control of the MPC to include the location of assistants, but the situation at least gives rise to the question of whether decisions about the employment of assistants take sufficient account of national manpower requirements.

3 The distribution of principals

> Where are the designated areas? I just always think of Birmingham.
>
> GP in Wiltshire
>
> Lord knows. In Wigan, I suppose.
>
> GP in Sussex

The analysis in the previous chapter was concerned with trends at the national level. Before moving on to consider the results of our survey of general practitioners the background information must be completed by examining patterns of distribution in each part of the country. At 1 January 1970 a fifth of all medical practice areas were designated, containing some 6,500 family doctors and over 18 million patients. Where were they located, and which suffered the greatest shortage of doctors? In attempting to answer this question the chapter deals first with the issue of selecting appropriate techniques of measurement; next it applies these measurements to the standard regions, geographical counties and executive councils; and finally it assesses the concentration and persistence of under-doctored areas in certain parts of the country.

Methods of measurement

The two alternative concepts of a fair distribution of doctors, described in Chapter 2, are reflected in two different ways of contrasting the shortage of manpower in different localities. The *spread* or extensiveness of the designated areas can be measured simply by counting the number of doctors practising in designated areas in each standard region, county, or whatever area unit is chosen. The variations between the units can then be assessed. Alternatively, the relative *depth* of deprivation in different places can be measured by calculating the number of extra doctors that would be needed in order to bring the average list size of the unit to 2,500. This figure may be expressed either as a *shortage* of GPs (when the average list exceeds 2,500) or as a *surplus* (when the average is less than 2,500).

Whichever of the two methods is used, it is generally desirable to express the results as rates rather than absolute numbers because the established area units (such as standard regions, executive councils, etc.) vary enormously in size. In 1970, for example, Lancashire Executive Council contained 509 principals in designated areas whereas Cambridgeshire and Isle of Ely Executive Council had only 11. These absolute numbers may be relevant for some purposes: they show, for instance, that however large a proportion this might represent of all principals in Cambridgeshire, the contribution of that executive council to the national situation was negligible. But for the purposes of *contrasting* the two executive councils these absolute numbers are useless: they must obviously be expressed as a proportion of all principals in each place. Similarly, the shortage (or surplus) of doctors can be expressed usefully as a rate per million patients.

It should be emphasised again that the two approaches do not necessarily yield consistent results. Depending upon internal variability, it is possible for an area unit to have an average list of less than 2,500 (and therefore suffer no shortage of doctors in terms of the second criterion) yet still to contain a fairly high proportion of practitioners in designated areas. The Newcastle Executive Council is a case in point: in 1970 this unit had an average list size of only 2,419, yet more than three-quarters (76 per cent) of all its principals were working in designated areas. The explanation lies in the heterogeneity within the unit whereby large lists in one practice area were offset for the purposes of calculating the average list size for the executive council by smaller lists elsewhere. The reverse situation, of units with a large shortfall of doctors but no designated areas, is much less common because it would require several areas with average lists well above 2,500 to remain for some reason undesignated.

Neither of these two ways of measuring the shortage of family doctors is inherently 'correct'. In general, the larger the unit the less useful is the second measure of shortfall, for large and significant local variations within the unit may be concealed within the overall average. On the other hand, by calculating the rate of shortfall (or surplus) it is possible to distinguish units requiring *extra* doctors in order to eliminate their designated areas from those which could achieve the same result merely by an internal redistribution of existing practitioners. Whenever there is a surplus it is always possible in principle to eliminate all designated areas in that unit merely by rearranging existing doctors, regardless of the actual proportion of

GPs in designated areas. Moreover, even among units which do actually require extra doctors, some need a good deal more than others. This can be put the other way round by saying that for the addition of a given number of doctors, many more people might be brought within list sizes of 2,500 in one unit than in another. It raises again the question of whether a redistributive policy (assuming it were effective) should seek primarily to achieve very substantial reductions in the average list sizes of a small number of heavily under-doctored areas, or to secure the greatest possible number of patients on lists below 2,500 (which would entail smaller reductions across a much larger number of areas).

It should by now be apparent that the choice of area units for the purpose of contrasting one part of the country with another is of considerable significance. For practical purposes the choice is limited to those units for which the appropriate statistics are available, namely standard regions, geographical counties and executive councils. Each of these units can be 'built up' of smaller units, but the relevant data are not always cumulative in the same way. A simple count of the number of doctors in designated areas *is* cumulative between each stage. For example, the number of 'designated doctors'[1] in the Northern region is the total of all such doctors in the five counties of the region, and the county totals are in turn the sum of all the designated doctors within each executive council. Figures of the shortfall of doctors in each unit are *not* cumulative in the same way, however, because larger units may conceal substantial differences between their constituent parts. Thus in the Northern region the average list size in 1970 was 2,528 and the absolute shortfall of doctors was 15. One or two of the counties in the region had quite large shortfalls, and the requisite number of extra doctors in order to bring the average list size in each *county* down to 2,500 was 65 – assuming, of course, that they were optimally distributed and that there was no movement of doctors from one county in the region to another. At the level of the executive councils the total shortfall was even greater (74), and although the figures for 1970 are not available it is probable that the summation by medical practice areas would have revealed an even higher total.

As this example demonstrates, the smaller the unit chosen the greater is the apparent total shortage of doctors. When the largest possible unit is taken (England as a whole) there was a small surplus in 1970 because the national average list was 2,478. By standard regions the shortfall was 275; by geographical counties it was 453; and by executive councils it totalled 527. The elimination of the designated areas thus depends to some extent upon the maximum area within which GPs are prepared to move and settle. If most doctors were willing to settle in any part of England then the problem would be simplified, for at the national level there are (just) enough GPs to eliminate all designated areas. Most doctors are evidently not as mobile as this, but they may, with an appropriate structure of incentives, be prepared to consider most places within any *region.* Some regions could then eliminate their designated areas by an internal redistribution without recourse to the influx of extra manpower. If, however, the *county* is the largest target area for doctors choosing a practice location then the relationship between redistribution and new resources shifts again. The ultimate question is: which geographical areas must achieve average lists below 2,500 for the problem to be considered solved? Current policy identifies the medical practice area as the critical unit, but the boundaries of these areas are arbitrarily determined and one of our conclusions in the final chapter is that they are inappropriate units by which to judge the adequacy of staffing levels.

The distribution of principals by standard regions[2]

Table A2 shows the proportion of principals in designated areas and the shortfall or surplus (as defined above) for each standard region and executive council in England at 1 October 1970. Corresponding figures for geographical counties are not given in the table because they can be calculated from the executive council figures, and data for individual medical practice areas are likewise not shown, partly because they are far too numerous and partly because the most recent available figures relate to 1967, since when the local situation has changed enormously.

Looking first at the eight standard regions, there were large differences between the regions in the proportions of principals practising in designated areas. The West Midlands stood out very clearly as the most extensively designated region (66 per cent of all principals), followed by the North (57 per cent), Yorkshire/Humberside (50 per cent), the East Midlands (44 per cent) and the North-West (42 per cent). None of the three southern regions had more than a fifth of its principals in designated areas, and the South-West had fewer than a tenth (8 per cent). These figures reveal a clear north/south split: just over half (51 per cent) of all principals to the north of a line from the Wash to the Severn were in designated areas in 1970 compared with only 17 per cent to the south, and the gap has been steadily widening over the past few years.

The second index of comparison, that of relative shortfalls or surpluses, also showed a similar north/south split, for whereas all the northern and midland regions had varying degrees of shortages, the three southern regions each enjoyed a surplus. This means that whilst all the designated areas in the south could in principle have been eliminated by an optimum redistribution of manpower *within* each region, the northern and midland regions would have needed a total of 275 *extra* GPs to achieve a similar result. The two midland regions suffered the most intense deprivations of manpower: not only were they extensively designated, they also experienced high shortfalls of doctors per million patients (−16·6 and −14·8 in the West and East Midlands respectively). The North-West had the next largest shortfall (−12·2 per million patients), followed by Yorkshire/Humberside (−7·8) and the North (−4·5). Of the three southern regions, the South-East had a more modest surplus (+12·0) than either East Anglia (+28·0) or the South-West (+46·4). In sum, the overall regional picture is one of an increasing relative shortage of family doctors as one moves from the Scottish border to the midlands, with a relative abundance to the south of the Wash–Severn line, especially towards the south-west.

The distribution of principals by executive councils

Because data relating to large geographical units may well conceal significant variations between sub-areas of the units, it is now necessary to look beyond the broad regional comparisons to more subtle local differences. The effect is analogous to that in microscopy, when the degree of magnification is increased and new shades and contours spring into view where formerly there had been only an area of apparent uniformity. It is, however, clearly impossible to cover the entire country in one short section, and we have therefore chosen to concentrate on six major clusterings of counties which in 1970 were both extensively designated and also experienced relatively large shortfalls of doctors.

The first cluster consists of the geographical counties[3] of Warwickshire and Staffordshire, which between them comprise ten executive councils and in 1970 contained 1,198 principals in designated areas – almost a fifth of all such doctors in the country. Three-quarters of them were concentrated in dense urban areas, with Birmingham, Coventry, Stoke and Wolverhampton accounting for more than half. Seven of the ten executive councils were wholly designated, and all had average list sizes above 2,500. The greatest shortages of principals, relative to size, were felt in Walsall, Wolverhampton, Stoke and West Bromwich: Birmingham itself, though still suffering an average list in excess of 2,500, had a shortage rate five times lower than that of Walsall.

The second cluster, in the East Midlands, is made up of the geographical counties of Derbyshire, Leicestershire and Nottinghamshire, and incorporates five executive councils. These counties in 1970 contained 473 principals in designated areas, almost half of all principals in the three counties and 7 per cent of all the designated doctors in England. A little over half of these 473 doctors were practising in the county boroughs of Nottingham, Derby and Leicester; the remainder were in the county areas. All five executive councils had average lists above 2,500, and the total shortfall of principals at executive council level was 53. Relative to size, the greatest shortages were felt in the three county boroughs, but even these rates were not as high as in many of the boroughs in Warwickshire and Staffordshire.

The third cluster appears in the South-East, and is made up of the counties of Essex, Hertfordshire, North-East London, and South-East London/Kent. (The latter two are, strictly speaking, executive councils rather than geographical counties.) These four counties, comprising five executive councils, contained a total of 1,003 principals in designated areas in 1970, equivalent to 47 per cent of all principals in the four counties or 16 per cent of all designated doctors in England. On the basis of the admittedly dated figures relating to medical practice areas (1967), three main concentrations of heavily designated localities are seen within these counties: one corridor stretching out from London through Essex, another group around the Luton–Watford area, and a third in the Medway towns. All five executive councils had average lists above 2,500 in 1970, and the total shortfall of principals at the executive council level was 64. Relative to size, the greatest shortages were felt in Hertfordshire and Essex, but, as in the East Midland cluster, these rates fell far short of those in the West Midlands or the North-East.

The fourth cluster, Lancashire, consists of the administrative county and seventeen county boroughs, each representing a separate executive council. Together they contained 925 principals in designated areas in 1970: 46 per cent of all principals in the county and 14 per cent of all designated doctors in the country. Not surprisingly, the administrative county contained the majority of these GPs, followed by eleven towns or cities with fewer than 100 each. It is interesting that in 1970 seven boroughs contained no designated areas at all, whilst neighbouring towns, apparently of similar composition, had quite large concentrations. In Manchester, for example, 21 per cent of principals were in designated areas and in the nearby towns of Bolton, Bury, Oldham and Rochdale the percentage was 100; yet in Salford, which virtually begins in the centre of Manchester, no areas were designated, and the second major Lancashire city (Liverpool) was also free of such areas. Twelve of the eighteen executive councils in the county had average lists above 2,500, and the total shortfall of principals at executive council level was 110. Standardised to population size, the greatest shortages were in Rochdale and St Helens (among the highest anywhere in the country), Bury, Blackburn and Bolton.

The fifth cluster, the West Riding of Yorkshire, consists of the administrative county and eleven county boroughs, each representing a separate executive council. Together they contained 793 principals in designated areas in 1970, equivalent to 53 per cent of all principals in the county and 12 per cent of all designated doctors in the country. About two-fifths of these 793 GPs were practising in the administrative county, Sheffield contained 147 of them, and eight other towns or cities had fewer than 100 each. Only two boroughs, Dewsbury and York, had no designated areas at all, and these were also the only two with average lists below 2,500. The total shortfall of principals at executive council level was 62, and the highest rates of shortfall were experienced in Rotherham and, to a lesser degree, Sheffield, Bradford and Halifax.

The sixth cluster is made up of the geographical counties of Durham and Northumberland, and incorporates nine executive councils. They contained 571 principals in designated areas in 1970, exactly two-thirds of all principals in the two counties and just under a tenth of all the designated doctors in England. The county areas of Durham accounted for 211 of these GPs, Newcastle and Sunderland together accounted for a further 161, and the remainder were distributed through all the other executive councils except Gateshead. This latter borough, together with Newcastle and Northumberland county, had an average list size below 2,500 in 1970; all the others had varying degrees of manpower shortage. The total shortfall of principals at the executive council level was 55, and the towns most affected, relative to size, were Hartlepool (with the highest average list size in the country), Darlington, Sunderland, Tynemouth and Durham.

These six clusters of counties contained between them more than three-quarters of all English-based principals in designated areas in 1970, and they represent those parts of the country which, on both measures of deprivation, were experiencing the most severe manpower difficulties. It should not be overlooked that many other counties also contained at least a few designated areas, some of them in seemingly unlikely places. Among areas which were designated in 1970 are: Maidenhead, Berkhamsted, Elstree, Potters Bar, Banbury, Highgate, Enfield, Bexley, Orpington, Tonbridge, Surbiton and Dover. Yet it remains generally true that the south was far less extensively designated than either the midlands or the north, for of the fourteen geographical counties in 1970 with fewer than 10 per cent of principals in designated areas only two (Herefordshire and Westmorland) lay to the north of the Wash–Severn line, and of the twenty-three counties with average lists below 2,500 only eight lay to the north. Counties with the greatest manpower problems were situated mainly around a line drawn from Kent to Lancashire, with an intensification in the midland counties and, away from the line, in the north-east. Counties to the west of a line from about Eastbourne to Chester had problems neither of depth nor of extensiveness (with the exception of Worcestershire), and the same can be said of East Anglia and most of the northernmost counties.

The concentration and persistence of designated areas

We conclude this chapter with a review of the evidence of the spatial and temporal persistence of designated areas. One possible form of spatial concentration is in large urban areas, and an indication was given in the previous section of the extent to which this was happening in the six clusters. By calculating for each geographical county the proportions of *all* principals and *designated* principals practising in county boroughs it is possible to draw some very broad conclusions about the urban/rural distribution of designated areas across the country as a whole. The resulting picture is not completely accurate for in some cases the executive council statistics for a county borough cannot be separated from its surrounding county (e.g. Nottingham, Oxford, Luton and Canterbury), and Greater London must for this purpose be treated as five county boroughs, corresponding with the five London executive councils. With these reservations in mind, the results show that in 1970 51 per cent of *all* principals and 55 per cent of *designated* principals in England were practising within the county boroughs. The slight excess of designated doctors in the county boroughs is insufficiently great to support the conclusion that the problem of under-doctored areas is overwhelmingly one of the large towns and cities. However, the Greater London area has an important distorting effect, for if the figures are reworked to *exclude* the London executive councils the remaining boroughs contained 48 per cent of the designated doctors but only 36 per cent of all principals.

Outside the capital, therefore, the under-doctored areas *were* more heavily concentrated in the large towns than would be expected on a purely random basis, and the annual reports of the Ministry of Health indicate that this has been the case at least since 1954. Of individual counties in 1970, Cumberland, Lincolnshire, Norfolk, Worcestershire and the East Riding had more than twice the expected proportion of designated GPs in the boroughs, and the proportion was at least one-and-a-half times greater in Derbyshire, Gloucestershire, Northumberland and the North Riding. By contrast, the counties of Devonshire, Hampshire, Northamptonshire, Somerset, Suffolk and Sussex had no designated doctors at all in their county boroughs. In sum, in spite of the possibility of fairly large annual fluctuations, the extent to which the under-doctored areas are concentrated in a predominantly urban environment depends not only upon the way in which an area is defined, but also upon the part of the country in question. Over the country as a whole doctors in designated areas are slightly over-represented in the county boroughs, but if London is excluded the tendency becomes much more marked.

Evidence for the persistence of under-doctored areas over time is of three kinds. On a long-term perspective the situation in 1970 can be compared with the pre-NHS distribution of practitioners revealed in the 1944 PEP Broadsheet which contained a map showing the location of doctors, by counties, in 1938. The overall impression is that the basic patterns have remained largely unaltered over the past thirty years. In 1938, as in 1970, there was a marked lack of doctors in the Midlands, Lancashire and Durham, with a relative abundance in the South, particularly the South-West. But in some detailed respects the emphasis has changed somewhat over this period. In 1938, for example, Warwickshire seemed to have a lower average list size than the other counties in the East and West Midlands, although it is difficult from the original map to make an accurate allowance for Birmingham. The northern home counties also seemed to be rather better off pre-war, for there is no sign in the 1938 map of the serious shortage of doctors which now besets north-east London and Hertfordshire, and to a lesser extent Bedfordshire, Buckinghamshire, and Essex. By contrast, it is clear that Sussex, like Westmorland, has never had any difficulty in attracting and retaining an adequate supply of family doctors. To this extent, at least, the National Health Service has not brought about any dramatic shift in the location of GPs, and the apparent chronicity of the problem in many places suggests that easy or quick solutions are unlikely to be found.

The second kind of evidence is to be found in trends in individual executive councils since the inception of the NHS. The councils fall into three categories: those with persistent histories of large lists (i.e. above 2,500), those which have never had large lists, and those which have sometimes experienced large lists. In the first category are the executive councils of Bedfordshire, Derbyshire, Durham, Essex, Lancashire, Lincolnshire, Staffordshire, Nottinghamshire, Warwickshire, Barnsley, Coventry, Dudley, St Helens, Sunderland, West Bromwich, and Wolverhampton. Almost all of these councils had high proportions of doctors in designated areas and large shortfalls of practitioners in 1970, and most were in one of the six clusters of heavily under-doctored counties. Among the second category of councils (those which have never experienced large lists) are the executive councils of Cambridgeshire, Cornwall, Cumberland, Devon, Dorset, Gloucestershire, Hampshire, Herefordshire, Norfolk, Oxfordshire, Somerset, Suffolk, Surrey, Sussex, Westmorland and the North Riding of Yorkshire. Each of these counties had a surplus of family doctors in 1970 and most had no designated areas. Again, this suggests that places with few manpower problems in 1970 have generally been able to attract sufficient doctors to keep their average list sizes below the figure for the country as a whole. The third category of councils (those which have sometimes been short of doctors) is in many ways the most interesting for it shows how individual counties have fared in relation to national trends. In some cases the shortage is of quite recent origin and probably attributable more to the movement of population than to the movement of doctors. Berkshire, for example, did not appear in the list until 1964, and Hertfordshire, Leicestershire, Cheshire and Wiltshire were all absent until 1958. Other counties have a less consistent history, being in the list some years and out of it in others. They include Huntingdonshire, South-West London, Northamptonshire, Middlesex and Worcestershire. Of the county boroughs, Gateshead, Great Yarmouth, Norwich, Southampton, Wigan, York and Birkenhead all had fairly large lists until about 1963 and then appeared to reduce them, whilst Burton, Dewsbury, Hartlepool, Tynemouth, Stoke, Walsall, Worcester, Blackburn, Oldham and Hull have only appeared in the list since that date.

The third kind of evidence of the temporal persistence of under-doctored areas lies in regional trends since the introduction of the designated area allowance in 1966. Has the recent pause in the spread of the designated areas, noted in Chapter 2, been felt equally in all parts of the country, or have some regions benefited at the expense of others? During the period between 1968 and 1970 the proportion of all principals in designated areas in England fell very slightly, but only two of the eight regions experienced a similar decline: the East Midlands, where the proportion fell from 59 to 44 per cent, and the South-East, with a drop from 24 to 20 per cent. In the remaining six regions the proportions rose: in East Anglia by 9 per cent, and elsewhere by between 1 and 4 per cent. The arrest in the spread of designated areas in the last year or two has therefore been confined principally to a couple of regions only, with little or no change in other parts of the country. Moreover, the sheer size of the South-Eastern region means that on a simple north/south split the south is being de-designated at a faster rate than the north. The widening disparity in the proportions of principals in designated areas is further evidence of this tendency.

In sum, we conclude from these analyses that the broad patterns of staffing needs have not changed dramatically over the last twenty to thirty years. Areas which are currently facing the most serious shortages seem to have a fairly long history of manpower difficulties, whilst those which are today relatively well supplied with family doctors have generally had no difficulty in past years in attracting and keeping an adequate number of practitioners. This conclusion suggests that there is unlikely to be any easy or quick solution to the problem of the unequal distribution of general practitioners.

4 A survey of general practitioners

I don't like people who do surveys.

GP in Worcestershire

The first three chapters utilised existing information to sketch in some of the historical dimensions to the problem of under-doctored areas and to describe trends in the distribution of family doctors. The aim has been to define the nature of the problem underlying the research with greater precision, and to clarify some of the conceptual and methodological issues involved in policy decisions. Our attention must now turn to the questions of why inequalities in distribution arise in the first place, how they are maintained, and what can be done about them. How often do GPs change practices and what is the relationship of mobility potential to career and family development? Which areas gain and lose in the net balance of migration? What relationship does the choice of a practice area have with a doctor's family home area, the location of his medical school and the family ties of his wife? What features distinguish doctors in designated areas from those elsewhere? What perceptions do GPs in different areas have of the professional, social and cultural value of their neighbourhoods? What do they think about the designated area allowances?

Answers to such questions are not to be found in official statistics; they can come only from a study of family doctors themselves. While general practice must be among the most intensively surveyed of British professions, very little relevant data already exist. Most surveys have been local rather than national, and none of the nation-wide surveys has elicited residential mobility and settlement patterns in the detail required by this study. Of the national surveys, Cartwright's study of doctors and their patients in 1964 can be analysed by type of practice area, but her schedule contained no questions relating specifically to the choice of practice area.[1] Last's surveys in 1967 and 1970 of regional patterns of settlement of doctors in relation to their home areas and medical schools are more closely related to the objectives of the current study than any other British survey, but the questionnaire was short and the results lack detail.[2,3] Of the local investigations, the most important is that undertaken by Brown and Walker in three areas based on Hull, Cardiff and Southampton.[4,5] An extensive literature exists of mobility and migration patterns in general populations[6] and also among medical practitioners in other countries,[7] but it was clear from an early stage that the information needed for this particular research could be obtained only through a specially designed survey. This chapter describes the main features of the survey design.

The sample

Various factors influenced the definition of the population and the size of the sample, including the desirability that it be widely distributed over the country, the need for an adequate number of doctors in each region and type of area, the availability of a central national sampling frame, and the possibility (not finally confirmed at the time of drawing the sample) that the survey might be conducted through the post. In the event, the population consisted of all unrestricted principals contracted with executive councils in England, and the sample was drawn in such a way that it would be suitable either for a postal survey or, in reduced form, for an interview survey. Wales was excluded because its small number of designated areas (only five in 1968, when the research was being planned) would have yielded a low pay-off in relation to the extra cost and complexity of extending the research there. Likewise Scotland had only eighteen designated districts in mid-1968, and has the added difficulty of an entirely separate system of administration, finance and record-keeping. The sample, drawn from the Doctor Index held by the Department of Health and Social Security, was originally correct at 1 October 1967, but later, when the revised Index became available in 1969, it was updated to October 1968. Since the survey itself was conducted between November 1969 and February 1970 there was a slight but inevitable incompleteness in the sample by comparison with the population of GPs at the time of the survey. Conversely, some doctors originally drawn in the sample were found to have died or retired after the survey began.

The population was stratified by standard region and type of practice area (that is, whether designated or non-designated). The original sampling goal was a target of about 2,000 doctors using a systematic one-in-eight sampling fraction in the designated areas in each region and a one-in-ten fraction in the non-designated areas. In the event, however, these fractions were amended to include all designated doctors in East Anglia and the South-West (since there were not many of them) and to provide a minimum of 100 non-designated practitioners in each region. Strictly speaking, therefore, the sampling fractions were not quite uniform within the designated/ non-designated strata over the regions. However, in view of the small numbers involved the analysis assumes uniform regional sampling fractions within each stratum, and very little precision is lost as a result. At this stage the sample amounted to 2,360 GPs, and it was reduced to 2,266 after up-dating to October 1968. The pilot survey consumed a further 100 doctors, and subsequent reductions due to death, retirement, etc. resulted in a final sample size of 2,031, of whom 816 were in designated areas and 1,215 in non-designated areas. A comparison of some characteristics of doctors in the sample with those of all principals in England and Wales in 1968 showed that the sample was very similar to the population in its distribution with respect to sex, age, classification of area, type of practice, and list size.

The pilot and main surveys

A small pilot survey was carried out in the summer of 1969 to test the adequacy of the questionnaire and to assess the merits of alternative methods of data collection. At the outset of the project two methods seemed feasible for the main survey: an interview survey conducted by the Regional Medical Officers (RMOs), or a postal survey. Both methods were used in the pilot survey and the results contrasted for differences in response rates and in the content of responses. One batch of fifty-three GPs received a postal questionnaire directly from the University of Kent and a second batch of forty-seven doctors was interviewed by RMOs in the Western, Southern and Eastern Divisions. The first batch yielded a response rate of 60 per cent without any follow-ups, and it was estimated that two follow-ups would have raised the final total to about 80 per cent. In the second batch the overall response was 84 per cent, and because of the large variations in response between the three divisions (ranging from 71 to 95 per cent) it was felt that the diligence of individual RMOs was possibly a critical factor. In both cases the response rates were similar for doctors in designated and non-designated areas, but a higher proportion of replies came from male doctors and from those with higher qualifications and larger lists. In view of the desirability of including as many doctors as possible it was decided that a postal survey would be the appropriate research tool in the main phase, but since the involvement of the Regional Medical Officers appeared to increase the motivation to respond it was also decided that the survey should be sponsored by the Divisional Medical Offices.

The first mailing in the main survey in November 1969 consisted of a seven-page questionnaire, a covering letter printed on the appropriate Divisional notepaper and signed personally by each doctor's Regional Medical Officer, and a reply-paid envelope addressed directly to the University.[8] Those who had not replied within about two weeks of the first mailing received a follow-up letter on University notepaper, signed by the senior research worker on the project and stressing the importance of achieving a high response rate. A second follow-up, consisting of a further questionnaire and reply envelope and another letter from the senior research worker was sent in February 1970 following a trial run in one division which amply showed the benefits which a third mailing would bring. The reply lists were closed in March 1970 when analysis of the data began, although the odd reply continued to come in right through to November.

Of the 2,166 doctors in the sample at the beginning of the survey, 135 were removed from the sample denominator as their circumstances were revealed: 20 had died; 83 had retired, resigned or, in one case, been struck from the Register; 24 could not be traced at all; and 8 were removed for special reasons (e.g. long-term hospital care) which meant that they were not actually practising as NHS principals at the time of the survey. This left 2,031 eligible respondents of whom almost two-thirds (64 per cent) replied to the first mailing (Table A3). The second mailing yielded a further 15 per cent of the total sample or just over two-fifths (43 per cent) of what was left; and the third mailing yielded another 6 per cent of the total, equivalent to 26 per cent of what remained at that time. In total, therefore, 1,721 usable replies were received, giving an overall response rate of 84·7 per cent. In designated areas the rate was 84·2 per cent and in non-designated areas it was 85·1 per cent. These responses are highly satisfactory and compare favourably with other recent national postal surveys of general practitioners.[9] There were no great variations in response either between divisions or even between executive councils. In thirty executive councils the response was 100 per cent whilst at the other extreme a handful of large executive councils had rates below 80 per cent, including Inner London, Liverpool, Walsall, Warwickshire and Birmingham. Response rates were generally higher in rural than in urban areas, and lowest in the large cities and conurbations of the country – London, Birmingham, Manchester and Liverpool. Proximity to London did not appear to be a factor in response although the rate for Inner London itself was low (68 per cent).

The sample print-out from the Doctor Index contained sufficient information about each GP to enable quite detailed comparisons to be made between respondents and non-respondents (Table A4). Five points of comparison are used: classification of practice area, sex, age, list size and number of principals in the practice. Despite the large numbers involved no statistically significant differences were observed between the actual frequencies and the expected frequencies calculated on the assumption that each attribute had no effect upon the probability of response. It can therefore be said with some confidence that those who returned their completed questionnaires were a satisfactory cross-section of all GPs in the sample. There were, however, some discrepancies at the extremes of some attributes, especially where the frequencies were low. Female doctors in designated areas were under-represented, and so too were elderly doctors and those with small list sizes in both designated and non-designated areas, but these latter two characteristics were highly associated with each other. No comparative information is available for the less tangible aspects of the quality of practice, and indeed there are hardly any such indicators that could be applied to non-respondents. Cartwright obtained a higher response from members of the Royal College of General Practitioners than from non-members, and also from doctors with post-graduate qualifications than from those with graduate or licentiate qualifications only (confirming our findings in the pilot survey). These results suggest that 'better' doctors (at least in terms of qualifications) may be relatively over-represented among respondents in postal surveys, but we have no systematic evidence from the present survey.

Coding and punching

The information from the questionnaires was coded onto IBM instruction sheets by a team of housewives, working part-time at home, who had already gained experience on other surveys. Each questionnaire was coded independently by two different coders, and double checks were made on the consistency of the two sets of codes.

The chief difficulties at this stage arose over the handling of unedited data. For reasons of time and cost it was decided to omit the editing stage and to pass the questionnaires for coding exactly as they were returned by the doctors. This meant that coders were often presented with material that was incomplete, ambiguous, inconsistent and often illegible, and in each case a decision was needed about handling it. The rule was therefore established that such queries were to be referred back to the supervisor or project director and all new decisions were immediately communicated to the coding team.

The total number of *detected* coding errors and discrepancies was at a rate of 0·6 errors per questionnaire or approximately 8 per 1,000 coding decisions. An error rate of this magnitude is well within the accepted limits of tolerance, and many of the recorded discrepancies were differences of opinion rather than outright errors. It is thus possible that the error rate in the strict sense was in fact lower than this. Against this, several hitherto undetected errors were discovered at the stage of data cleaning, and in addition all survey data inevitably contain a small proportion of undetected coding errors.

The data were punched onto 80-column cards, verified by machine, and cleaned on a counter-sorter. Cleaning involved checking that all codes were within the specified range for each variable and that all internal consistencies held good. Data were then transferred to tape for computer analysis.

The follow-up survey

A postal survey has certain strengths and weaknesses in comparison with other types of surveys. If the problem of low response can be overcome (which is the chief disadvantage of the method) a postal survey is usually much cheaper than any other form of data collection, but it has the added drawback of being limited mainly to simple factual questions. A mail questionnaire is not good at tapping opinions or attitudes, and complex questions requiring long written answers are best omitted. Much of the information needed in this study was of a type that could properly be collected through a postal survey, but it also seemed useful to supplement the responses with more subjective material for illustrative purposes. To this end a small follow-up survey was mounted in September 1970 in which semi-structured interviews were conducted with thirty of the original respondents and, where possible, with their wives also. These doctors were practising in areas of the country with very diverse manpower situations, and all had moved either from a designated to a non-designated area or vice versa. The interviews were tape-recorded and some of the material from them is presented in Chapter 12.

Presentation of the survey data

The fact that the research design effectively yielded two samples (one of doctors in designated areas and the other of those in non-designated areas) means that the results obtained from the two samples cannot strictly be aggregated to give representative results for the country as a whole. In most of the subsequent tables, therefore, the results are presented separately for the designated and non-designated samples. Where estimates are required for the *total* population of doctors (as for example in Chapter 6) they are obtained by weighting the designated and non-designated samples to take account of the differential sampling fractions. It should be noted in this context that the non-designated sample includes all doctors who, at the time of the survey, were practising in open, intermediate or restricted areas, although in many tables the results are listed separately for each individual type of area.

In most cases the figures presented in the tables are the raw sample frequencies, without adjustment for non-response and without inflation to population estimates. The decision to leave the sample frequencies unadjusted for non-response was based upon the fact that, as far as could be ascertained, the respondents were a representative sample of all doctors approached, and consequently the failure to achieve a 100 per cent response merely affected the size of the sample and not its representativeness with respect to the population of GPs. Population estimates are rarely given because in most tables the primary interest lies in contrasting the proportions of doctors in various categories possessing a relevant characteristic, but sample frequencies can quite easily be inflated if the reader wishes to do so. As a guideline, if 200 respondents in the designated sample had a certain attribute, then there is a 95 per cent chance that between 1,700 and 2,120 GPs in designated areas throughout England also possessed that attribute in 1968. For a designated sample frequency of 400 the population range lies between 3,590 and 4,050; and for a frequency of 600 the range is 5,570–5,880. Population ranges at 95 per cent confidence for sample frequencies in the non-designated sample are: for 300, 3,210–3,860; for 600, 6,720–7,420; and for 900,

10,360–10,840. The standard error of the percentage, with finite population correction, is calculated as:

$$\sqrt{\frac{pq}{n} \left[\frac{N-n}{N}\right]}$$

where N and n are respectively the population and sample sizes; p is the percentage of the sample possessing the characteristic in question; and q = (100−p). These limits are probably conservative as they assume simple random sampling, whereas the actual sampling scheme was systematic random with stratification by regions.

Lastly, significance tests are rarely given in the text or by the tables. The main reason for this is that significance tests in common use relate to an individual characteristic of a table or a result, whereas arguments in a research report of this kind tend to be based on a complex of results. In such cases it is more important to observe and explain a set of results which are consistent with the argument than to dwell on the significance of individual results to the exclusion of others in the complex. It is possible to apply more sophisticated multivariate techniques to test the significance of complex hypotheses, but as a first step it seems more appropriate to present results based on survey data which are reasonably clear and indisputable, since it is on these that policy-makers can most readily base their actions.

5 The mobility of general practitioners

> I think you should certainly put down roots. You get to know patients when you stay in one place, and when you get to know them you want to carry on looking after them. That's why we're doctors, isn't it?
>
> GP in Leicester

The number of family doctors in any area is the net result of gains from and losses to other stocks of medical manpower, and the number may be changed by enlarging the gains or diminishing the losses or both. In practice some movements appear to be more easily influenced than others, and, perhaps reflecting this, the postwar history of manpower policy shows that greater effort has generally been expended nationally and locally on stimulating the gains than on controlling the losses. The success that can reasonably be expected from any attempts to persuade doctors to move will however depend to a large extent upon the mobility potential of the profession as a whole. How often do GPs move, and when are they most likely to move? If it should be shown that only a small proportion of doctors normally change practices during the course of their careers, or that those who do so are mainly elderly practitioners seeking smaller practices for their last few years, then the implications would be different (and possibly more serious) than a situation in which most doctors moved at least once in their lives, and at a fairly young age.

This chapter is concerned with the extent to which the doctors in the survey had moved from practice to practice during their careers, and the circumstances under which they had done so. The analysis is complicated by the ambiguity of the concept of 'mobility' and also by the technical problems arising from the cross-sectional or 'once-off' nature of the survey. On the question of definition, the concept of mobility is used in two distinct ways. In one context it describes a career move from one practice to another. General practitioners do not always need to change practices to achieve career advancement: many are promoted from assistant to partner in the same practice and some may move immediately into general practice as principals. But for many doctors at least one move has been a necessary condition of advancement, particularly in the early years of the NHS when the number of assistants seeking partnerships far exceeded the number of vacant posts. Yet even a large number of moves by family doctors would not necessarily constitute a potential source of geographical redistribution, for most moves may prove to be local, within the boundaries of the same executive council or even the same medical practice area. The second usage of the concept of mobility is therefore in the geographical sense of movement from one area unit to another. The unit may be a standard region, county, executive council, medical practice area, or whatever is chosen as appropriate. Thus by definition geographical mobility always implies movement between practices, but the reverse may not hold good in the light of what is taken to be the appropriate unit for the purposes of assessing geographical mobility.

The second general difficulty underlying the analysis is that of allowing for the effects of time. Since the survey was a snapshot picture of a cross-section of GPs at a single moment in time, it included doctors scattered across the whole of the age range. Results based on total data for the two samples are consequently a sort of average of all trends over the past forty years or more, and may conceal important differences between generations. Mobility may have become much more or much less common since the inception of the NHS, in which case the more recent trends will be of the greatest interest. The best way of studying such trends is by following successive cohorts of doctors over a long period of time, but this approach is costly and time-consuming. In this study we have had to resort to the second-best alternative of reconstructing inter-generation variations within cross-sectional data. The method has certain imperfections. In particular, for each successive generation the upper age limit decreases in a cross-sectional survey, and the *completed* career patterns cannot strictly be compared. This problem is discussed in greater detail later in the chapter in relation to the actual results of the survey.

Mobility between practices

The doctors participating in the survey were asked to list all the positions they had ever held in general practice, except as locums. A change of position was defined as a move from one practice to a different one, and specifically excluded promotions within the same practice. Just over 40 per cent of family doctors in each sample were still working in the same practice in which they had started, and about a third had worked in two different practices (that is, they had moved once). The remainder, about a quarter, had held three or more different positions, which means that they had moved from one practice to another on at least two occasions. It seems on past experience that more than half of all general practitioners can expect to change practices at least once during their careers, although most of those who do move will do so only once. There were no great differences in this respect between doctors in each type of practice area except that those in restricted areas had made rather more multiple moves than the rest. A small list size, probably in a pleasant residential area, may be the reward of those prepared to make several moves. It was not uncommon in pre-NHS days for doctors to do a stint in industrial working-class districts before selling up and moving to a seaside or rural practice, and although the sale of practices is no longer legal the Medical Practices Committee has urged executive councils to give full consideration to doctors who, having spent much of their careers in heavy industrial areas, seek more modest vacancies in pleasanter places towards the end of their working lives.[1]

The important question surrounding these results is whether doctors entering general practice in recent years are likely to move more or less frequently than their older colleagues. The answer is complicated by the fact that there is in any case an obvious relationship between age and mobility: doctors who have worked in three or four different practices, for example, are not likely to be much under 35. So quite apart from any changes over time we would expect the younger respondents in the survey to have moved less often than the older ones, even though their eventual career mobility may prove to be higher. The critical question is whether, before settling down in their main life-time practice, younger doctors nowadays are more likely to move than their older colleagues did before *they* settled. The answer we can give is inevitably imperfect because many of the younger doctors in the survey had almost certainly not yet settled and there is no sure way of telling how often they will move before doing so. If, however, it is assumed for the time being that most GPs will have settled by the time they reach 40 it is at least possible to compare mobility patterns up to that age through to the late 1950s. In particular, since virtually all doctors under 50 at the time of the survey would have spent all their time as GPs within the National Health

Service, some simple comparisons can be made between the periods before and after 1948.

The figures in Table A5 confirm that the youngest doctors (those under 30) in both samples had indeed moved less frequently, on average, than their older colleagues. Those in the next two age groups (30–39) had made an intermediate number of moves, but among those over 40 there were no major differences in either sample. There is certainly no firm evidence that doctors starting in general practice before 1948 had been consistently more or less mobile than those who had practised exclusively within the NHS. Nevertheless there are some indications that younger GPs may change practices more often than doctors have done in the past. Those in the age group 40–44, for example, had already made as many moves, on average, as doctors in any of the higher groups, and over a lifetime they will probably make more moves. It is impossible to estimate the eventual mobility potential of the youngest doctors (under 35) with any degree of certainty because new factors such as the introduction of the designated area allowance distort the extrapolation of past trends, but at least their record so far is consistent with the hypothesis of greater professional mobility potential among younger doctors entering general practice since the early 1960s.

A further interesting point in Table A5 is that doctors in the 55–59 age group in both samples had moved less frequently than most other GPs over 40. This may be more than a chance result, for most of the respondents in this age group were completing their medical training between about 1935 and 1939, and would probably have served throughout the war in the armed forces. Consequently their average age on entering general practice was some four or five years higher than usual, and this, coupled with the desperate scramble for principalships in the years leading up to 1948 and the unwillingness to move once such a post had been secured, would reasonably account for their relative immobility. Other evidence of the unsettling effects of the war was found by Brown and Walker in their study of general practitioners in East Yorkshire, South Hampshire and Glamorgan.[2] Only 58 per cent of those graduating between 1940 and 1954 had settled in the area of their first choice, compared with 68 per cent of the pre-1940 and post-1954 graduates. The evidence is therefore consistent: doctors whose training was affected by the war were older than average on entering general practice, therefore less likely to have moved, and consequently less likely to have finished up in the area of first preference.

Geographical mobility

Although a majority of general practitioners move from one practice to another during the course of their career, fewer are geographically mobile – at least between regions and counties. About two-thirds of the respondents in each sample had so far spent their entire time as GPs in the same standard region, and most of those who had crossed regional boundaries had done so only once.[3] Fewer than one doctor in ten had practised in more than two different regions. The question of how much manpower each region has gained and lost as a result of these movements is dealt with in the next chapter, but the judgment might be offered on the basis of the present information that family doctors are a rather more itinerant group than has hitherto been supposed. In the light of many complaints during the past decade about the unwillingness of GPs to consider the potential delights of new pastures it comes as a mild surprise to discover that about a third of them have at some time made the move from one region to another, and that almost one in ten have done so at least twice. The differences between the older and younger doctors are predictable: those under 40 had made fewer inter-regional moves, on average, than their older colleagues, although their eventual lifetime record may prove to be greater. Doctors in their forties in both samples had already achieved more inter-regional moves than those in the higher age ranges, and the 55–59 age group again showed less inclination to switch from one region to another than those in either the preceding or subsequent age groups.

Movement between geographical counties followed a similar pattern: an increasing number of inter-county moves, on average, in successive age groups up to about 40; broadly similar trends beyond that age with the exception of doctors in the 55–59 age range; and only a small proportion of moves between three or more different counties. As expected, however, the actual number of doctors in each sample moving across county boundaries was somewhat greater than the number moving from one region to another (40 per cent compared with about 33 per cent). Nevertheless most of those who had moved geographically had done so inter-regionally, for four-fifths of all doctors crossing county boundaries had also changed regions in the process.

The different types of career and geographical mobility described above can be combined in the following way:

1. Doctors who had spent their entire careers to date in the same practice (no mobility).
2. Doctors who had changed practices within the same county (mobility within county).
3. Doctors who had moved between counties within the same region (mobility within region).
4. Doctors who had moved from one region to another (mobility between regions).

The distribution of respondents in each sample between these four categories of movement is given in Table A6, with doctors above and below the age of 40 separated out. Even allowing for the limitations of a cross-sectional survey, it seems that these figures are tolerably good indicators of the amount and type of movement that can be expected from most *existing* practitioners over the course of a full career, although the situation may well be changing. Quite apart from general developments (planned and unplanned) in the structure and administration of general practice, there is evidence in the survey that younger doctors may now be more willing or more able to move than their counterparts in previous years. Already, doctors in their forties had, on average, changed practices more often than the older GPs and the full life-time differential will probably be even greater. There can be less certainty about the mobility potential of younger doctors because they had completed an insufficiently large part of their careers on which to base reliable predictions, but at least their performance so far is consistent with the hypothesis of greater freedom of movement. The implications of these results for planning and policy-making is intriguing. It seems generally to have been assumed that GPs have a low propensity for change and movement, and that an important aim of any incentive must be to stimulate initial ideas about the desirability of change. In fact the main problem may be less one of getting doctors to move in the first place than of directing their natural mobility potential into the 'right' areas and, having got them there, of encouraging them to stay. The next step must therefore be to identify the circumstances under which doctors tend to move.

Correlates of mobility

Age

It seems reasonably clear from the evidence in Table A5 that most doctors who move do so in the early years of their careers, possibly before they acquire family commitments and while they are seeking to establish themselves. Most changes of practice, especially among the older doctors in the survey, were from assistant to principal status, and in many cases were made after only a few years in general practice. Once settled as partners it is expected that subsequent changes will be few, with such exceptions as married women moving with their husbands and older practitioners moving to smaller practices towards the end of their careers. In fixing more precisely the age span during which most GPs change from one practice to another, the problem again arises of using a cross-sectional study for what should ideally be a longitudinal analysis. Whilst the ages of doctors when they took up their current appointments are known, there can be no certainty that these will be their terminal jobs. Indeed, many of the younger GPs in the survey undoubtedly will change practices again, some of them several times. There is no perfect solution to this problem without resort to a much larger and more complex study, but a sufficiently good estimate can be made by assuming as a general rule that the older a doctor grows the less likely he is to move again. The question then is whether the proportion of movers who had started their present posts by any given age is the same for the younger as for the older respondents.

The figures in Table A7 are restricted to respondents who had changed practices at least once, and they relate age at the time of the survey with age at starting current appointments. It is clear that older doctors had, as a rule, moved into their current posts at a later age than the younger respondents. If, for instance, those in the highest age group (60+) make no further moves before they retire, then more than a quarter of them will have changed practices after the age of 40 and at least one in ten will have moved after 50. In the next lowest age group (50–59) the proportion moving after 40 falls to about one-fifth, and the effects of the war are seen again in the relatively low proportion of these doctors who had started in their current posts by the age of 30. Whether the *completed* career histories of the younger respondents will finally show a similarity to that of the over-60s is a matter for speculation. The data in Table A7 are at least consistent with the possibility of this happening, but it could equally well transpire that these younger doctors might suddenly put down roots and remain in one place for the rest of their lives.

Certain background factors are relevant in forming an opinion. The difficulties of achieving partnership status in the 1950s and the consequent tendency for doctors at that time to spend quite long periods as assistants are less likely to affect those entering general practice today. It is much easier for a younger man to become a partner and achieve quick financial parity in the 1970s than ten or fifteen years earlier, and hence the opportunities to settle at an earlier age are greater. Reinforcing this is the fact that early marriage tends to diminish the likelihood of moving (see below), and that as the age of marriage falls so an increasing number of GPs can be expected to settle by about their mid-30s. The 1966 Association for the Study of Medical Education (ASME) survey showed that of final-year medical students in that year 22 per cent were married and 14 per cent were either engaged or intending to be married within a year.[4] By 1971 the proportion of final-year students who were married had risen to about 25 per cent. Against this interpretation, however, is the earlier conclusion that the younger respondents showed clear signs of making at least as many career moves as their older colleagues had done, and perhaps even more. Unless they deviate radically from the mobility patterns of their immediate seniors it seems that the future tendency may be for doctors entering general practice to make one or two quick moves before settling at a comparatively young age. It would, however, clearly be desirable to know the extent to which this does in fact occur, and we return in the concluding chapter to the question of monitoring the movement of family doctors.

Marriage and family responsibilities

The evidence from the survey shows that the younger a doctor marries the less likely he is to move, even when allowance is made for the effect of his age. Respondents who had married *after* entering general practice were more mobile in every sense than those marrying *before* starting their careers as GPs: they were more likely to have changed practices, more likely to have done so several times, and more likely to have crossed regional boundaries. The differences are consistent in both samples. Even when the effect of age is controlled the significance of the timing of marriage remains. Of doctors over 40, for example, 46 per cent of those in the non-designated sample who had married before taking their first jobs in general practice were still in the same practice compared with only 36 per cent of those marrying after. In the designated sample the respective proportions were 41 per cent and 32 per cent. Among respondents under 40 the trends are naturally less clear, but they are consistent with the conclusion that early marriage has tended to reduce the likelihood of family doctors moving in the past, and it may still have this effect.

Part of the explanation lies not only in the marriage itself but also in the consequent assumption of family responsibilities. As a rule the younger people marry the earlier they assume the responsibilities of parenthood, and hence the timing of the marriage appears to be an indirect rather than a direct factor in mobility. It is in general easier for single people and childless couples to move house than for families, and unless the children are at boarding school the upheavals usually increase as the children get older. There is clear evidence from the survey that the decision to settle is closely related to the cycle of family development, and particularly to the educational needs of the children. Just over two-fifths of the married doctors had started in their current positions before they had any children, and over 90 per cent had started before the eldest child had reached secondary school age. Put the other way round, fewer than one married doctor in ten had so far moved *after* his eldest child had reached 11 years of age. Even among those who had moved more than once the proportions who had changed practices after their children had reached secondary school age were only 16 per cent and 11 per cent respectively in the designated and non-designated samples. With a few exceptions, therefore, doctors who had changed practices after the age of about 40 were either those who had never married (of whom there were very few in either sample) or those who were later in starting their families.

Post-graduate training

The results discussed so far suggest that events which postpone the age of entry into general practice also reduce mobility potential. This is a reasonable conclusion from the relationship between marriage and mobility, and the effect of the second world war has already been noted. Happily, war is epiphenomenal, and post-graduate training is a much more common reason for late entry into general practice. On the basis of the analysis so far we would expect that, other things being equal, GPs pursuing post-graduate training and higher degrees would be less likely to move than those who are not. The evidence confirms this to be the case, even when age is controlled. Among the over-40s in the designated sample, 46 per cent of those gaining secondary qualifications[5] before entering general practice had stayed in the same practice up to the time of the survey compared with only

29 per cent of those who obtained such qualifications after starting in practice. In the non-designated sample the corresponding percentages were 49 and 37. Doctors with no additional qualifications fell midway between these extremes in both samples. There remains the possibility that respondents who had gained their further qualifications before entering practice may have differed from the rest in other ways which affected their mobility potential, but the results are at least consistent with the basic hypothesis about the relationship between mobility and the career cycle.

Birthplace

The influence of certain biographical factors on a doctor's choice of practice location is considered in some detail in Chapter 7, but it is interesting at this point to contrast the experiences of English-born and non-English-born practitioners. It is difficult to predict whether those born outside the country may be more or less likely to change practices and move from one area to another than English-born doctors. On the one hand it is arguable that having already made one significant move (though not necessarily as a GP) they would be more disposed towards subsequent ones; on the other hand many respondents of foreign nationality reported considerable difficulties in obtaining the kind of practice they wanted, and several had been unable to move even when they wished to. The evidence from the survey is equivocal. Forty-one per cent of the designated sample and 34 per cent of the non-designated sample had been born outside England, most of them in Scotland or Ireland, and as a whole they had moved more frequently, and probably over a greater distance, than those born in England. In the designated sample, for instance, 35 per cent had remained in the same practice up to the time of the survey and 42 per cent had crossed regional boundaries, compared with 45 per cent and 30 per cent respectively among their English-born counterparts. Similar percentages are found in the non-designated sample. These results tend to support the argument that having made at least one international residential move people are less likely subsequently to settle in one place, but many other factors may be affecting the results. Moreover, the mobility patterns of doctors born in each individual country show much inconsistency, although the frequencies are admittedly low. It seems safe to conclude that GPs born outside England are likely to respond at least as favourably as English-born practitioners to incentives to move, although the reasons for this are unclear.

6 An area analysis of mobility patterns

> My wife and I would both like to move to the south of England.
>
> GP in Lancashire

In this chapter the analysis of mobility patterns is carried one stage further by considering how they have affected different parts of the country. The point was made in Chapter 2 that the number of principals in any locality is eventually determined by offsetting the gains of GPs from different sources against the losses incurred for various reasons. Incoming doctors may include those entering general practice for the first time, those coming into the country from abroad, and those moving from practices elsewhere in the country. Losses may result from death, retirement, resignation etc., as well as from doctors moving out to practices in other parts of the country. It is probable that most areas, over a period of time, will experience a mixture of these different forms of losses and gains, but the composition of the mixture may vary significantly from area to area and may even constitute a major factor in current manpower shortages. If the 'performance' of different area units on each of these movements could be assessed and contrasted with the average performance for that unit across the country as a whole, then it would be possible to identify the main reasons why some areas suffer a shortage of family doctors. For example, in a county which would currently have an average list size below 2,500 had it been able to attract the same proportion of doctors entering general practice for the first time as most other counties, the remedy for the manpower shortage might be sought in more vigorous publicity among younger doctors and medical students. In another case the major deficit may be of doctors entering the country from abroad or moving from other areas, or the shortage may lie in abnormally high wastage rates through death or retirement.

A full analysis of this kind would be exceedingly complicated, and would require longitudinal data. It would enable us to take a particular unit and a particular starting date and then trace the gross gains and losses to the unit over any chosen time period. The results could be presented in the form that between one date and another the unit had recorded a gross gain of x practitioners (made up of such-and-such a proportion of newly qualified doctors, immigrants from abroad, and family doctors moving from other parts of the country), and suffered a gross loss of y doctors (so many of whom died, retired, emigrated, or moved elsewhere). The individual doctors making up the results would change over the period under review as some came and some went, and there would probably be no single point in time when all the individuals in the analysis were practising together. A cross-sectional design, by contrast, *is* limited to just such a single moment of time, and hence any reconstruction of earlier migration patterns can take account only of those people in the system *at the one point in time*. It is possible from cross-sectional data to categorise the sources from which *existing* doctors in any unit derived, but there can be no record of those who came and then died or retired or moved elsewhere before the survey was made. The only losses revealed by such a study are those resulting from internal migration to other parts of the country, and they show up in the data as gains to the host area.

This point of methodology has been elaborated in some detail because the aim of this chapter is necessarily limited, and might easily be misunderstood. Our purpose is to reconstruct the geographical mobility patterns of a sample of doctors still in practice at the time of the survey, and then to use the results to see the extent to which the current manpower problems in an area may be attributable to adverse trends within those patterns. In doing this, the analysis around which the chapter is structured simply compares the *first* and the *current* practice locations of the doctors in the sample: the data cannot therefore indicate total changes in the stock of GPs in an area during a specified period of time. Such data, as we have explained, can be derived only from a longitudinal study. This limitation means that words such as 'gains' and 'losses' acquire a particular and somewhat restricted meaning. To say that a certain region has gained 150 GPs does *not* mean that a total of 150 practitioners had moved into the region during a specified time period: it means that 150 doctors *in the sample* were practising in that region *at the time of the survey*, having moved into it as GPs at some time in the past. Likewise to say that a certain county has lost 50 GPs means that 50 respondents in the survey had their first appointments in general practice in the county, but were currently practising elsewhere in England at the time of the survey. Similarly the phrase 'the number of doctors first practising in a region' does not refer to the total stock of GPs at some specific point in the past, but to the number of practitioners in the sample whose first appointment had been in that region. In short, our concern is with patterns of geographical mobility within a closed system, and with the extent to which these internal movements have affected the overall distribution of manpower.

In order to simplify what might easily become an impossibly complicated analysis the chapter concentrates on migration between standard regions[1] and between geographical counties. To confine the analysis to these two levels is to remain removed from the unit of ultimate significance (the medical practice area, since it is this unit which is either designated or non-designated), and certain assumptions must therefore be made about interchanges at the sub-county level. However, the results would not only become very complex if extended to executive councils and medical practice areas, but would also be of dubious value in many instances because the sample frequencies become very small. The main emphasis of the chapter is therefore on inter-regional migration, with some consideration given to the inter-county patterns. It is hoped that the results will at least give an indication of the value to be derived from a continuous monitoring of the geographical movements of family doctors.

Migration patterns: the net regional balance

Table A8 sets out the basic migration data at regional level. The figures in this and subsequent tables in the chapter are 1968 population estimates for England, obtained by inflating the sample frequencies by the appropriate factor for the designated and non-designated samples in each standard region. The first column shows the total number of principals practising in England in 1968 classified by their region of *first* practice (which in many cases, of course, is also their region of current practice), and expressed in column 2 as a base of 100. The total in this first column (17,309) is somewhat less than the full number of principals in 1968 because some had their first appointments outside England. Column 11 shows the distribution of principals in England in 1968 classified by their *current* region of practice at the time of the survey. The difference between the total in this column and the total in the first column is accounted for by doctors who had come in from outside England (column 9). The last column in the table expresses the numbers in column 11 as percentages of the numbers first practising in the regions.

Looking first at the overall changes recorded in columns 11 and 12, two regions (Yorkshire/Humberside and the South-West) have suffered a net loss of doctors of 4 per cent and 9 per cent respectively. This means that the net result of balancing the outward movement of doctors first practising in these two regions against the inflow of GPs from other regions and countries has been a loss of almost 70 practitioners from Yorkshire and about 170 from the South-West. These losses are more serious for Yorkshire than for the South-West, for even though the latter region has suffered the greater depletion of manpower it nevertheless remains well supplied with GPs. The projected rate of population growth is higher in the South-West, however, and it would be desirable to monitor future movements into and out of the region to identify the factors which may underlie any future increases occurring in list sizes in the region.

The West Midland region has broken even: that is, the gross gains to the region from various sources have been offset almost exactly by the losses. This region, however, is expected to be among the fastest growing regions over the next fifteen years, and it must either attract an increasing number of doctors or hold on to a greater proportion of them if the supply is to keep pace with population growth. The Northern region has experienced a net gain of some 70 principals (6 per cent). The regional average list size has been hovering around 2,500 for several years, and its projected rate of population growth is the lowest in the country. This is therefore a region in which one might look for no more than a moderate rate of increase in the stock of GPs. East Anglia has experienced a somewhat larger net percentage increase (11 per cent). At present the region is generally well supplied with family doctors, but it is expected to be the fastest growing region in the country over the next fifteen years, and it must continue to attract and retain practitioners in order to keep pace with the anticipated rapid population growth.

The South-East has shown a similar overall increase to East Anglia (12 per cent), but this region has almost reached its maximum expansion capacity for several years, and is expected to have a lower rate of population growth over the next fifteen years than any region except the North. The North-West, with a net gain of almost 20 per cent, has been one of the most successful regions in this respect, but it still has an average list above the 2,500 mark, and is expected to experience a moderately high rate of population growth in the short-term. Lastly, the East Midlands has shown a higher net percentage increase than any other region (26 per cent), but has still been unable to keep pace with the increase in population. The regional average list size has been rising steadily over the past few years, and the high projected rate of population growth makes it probable that the regional shortfall of doctors will continue at least for several years.

The balance of internal regional migration

These results suggest that the net regional gains and losses are unrelated to the current staffing situation in the regions. Although conclusions based upon only eight comparisons are necessarily tentative, there is no relationship between the magnitude of net gains and losses and the current surplus or shortfall of GPs at the regional level. The analysis must therefore focus upon the components of this overall situation, starting with the results of the *internal* movement of doctors within the country from one region to another. The figures are contained in columns 7 and 8 of Table A8, and since the gains to some regions are the losses from others, the sum total of such gains and losses is zero.

The regions fall roughly into four pairs. The first, comprising the South-East and East Anglia, both gained from the balance of internal movement (by 4 per cent and 5 per cent respectively), but would still have had regional average list sizes below 2,500 in 1968 *even if the balance had been zero.* Part of this gain has therefore been 'unnecessary' in the sense that it has diverted manpower to these regions which might be more urgently needed elsewhere. The 'unnecessary' migration routes are shown in Table A9. Reading across the rows, it is seen that the major sources of 'surplus' manpower into the South-East were the South-West, the North, Yorkshire/Humberside and the West Midlands; and the largest gains to East Anglia were from the North-West and South-West.

The second pair of regions, the East Midlands and the North-West, also gained from the balance of internal movement (by 16 per cent and 10 per cent respectively), but unlike East Anglia and the South-East their average list sizes were already in excess of 2,500 in 1968 and would have been even higher but for the gains. However, Table A9 shows that much of the increase in the East Midlands was at the expense of the West Midlands, and in the North-West at the expense of Yorkshire/Humberside and the West Midlands. It is therefore largely self-defeating since these two losing regions themselves suffered a shortfall of family doctors in that year.

The third pair of regions, the South-West and the North, both suffered a *loss* through internal migration (of 17 per cent and 5 per cent respectively), yet still managed to maintain a regional average list size below 2,500 in 1968. In the South-West, which lost most of its migrating doctors to the South-East and the West Midlands, the list size remained well below this figure. The situation in the Northern region is different, for although the percentage loss was much lower than in the South-West the regional list size had been hovering just below the 2,500 mark for some years prior to 1968, and exceeded it in 1969 and 1970. Most of those leaving this region went to the South-East and the North-West.

The last two regions, Yorkshire/Humberside and the West Midlands, also suffered a loss through the balance of internal migration (of 11 per cent and 7 per cent respectively) and in addition they had moderately large shortfalls of principals in 1968. These two regions have consequently suffered the most as a result of internal migration. The majority of GPs leaving Yorkshire went across the Pennines to the North-West, and some went to the South-East and the West Midlands. The greatest losses from the West Midlands were to the East Midlands, the South-East and the North-West.

The components of the balance of internal regional migration: gross losses

In the preceding two sections we considered the *net* changes in the manpower stock of each region resulting from the balance of all movements (including those into the country from outside as well as those internal to the country) and the balance of internal migration only. Already these results contain some interesting implications. It is seen from Table A9, for example, that the net effect of all movements of doctors between the South-East and Yorkshire/Humberside resulted in a loss to the latter region of about 40 practitioners – just a little more than the current total shortfall in the region shown in Table A2.[2] Bearing in mind that all these practitioners were 'surplus' to the requirements of the South-East, it follows that had the loss of doctors through this route alone been stemmed, the average list size in Yorkshire/Humberside in 1970 would have been below the 2,500 mark *without* raising it above this level in the South-East. The exercise can be repeated for each region, with variable conclusions. But before any final conclusions can be drawn about the relationship between mobility patterns and manpower distribution the analysis must focus still more finely upon the gross movements which together make up the balance of internal regional migration. We start with the gross losses (columns 3 and 4 in Table A8). Table A10 shows how the gross movement has affected each region in relation to every other region.

Some of the regions have lost more doctors through internal migration than others. In four regions (Yorkshire/Humberside, the East and West Midlands and the South-West) at least 30 per cent of doctors first practising there had subsequently moved out, compared with fewer than 20 per cent moving from the South-East and the North-West. There are clearer signs here of a link between past mobility and the current supply of medical manpower, for apart from the South-Western region those with the highest gross percentage losses generally had the greatest shortfalls of GPs. It seems possible that the contemporary shortage of family doctors in certain regions of the country may lie primarily in the failure to retain doctors who have once practised there rather than in the inability to attract them in the first place. This possibility is reinforced by a closer examination of the data, for if the regions with a shortage of doctors in 1968 had each been able to retain enough of those GPs who had moved to the three southern regions to ensure that their average list sizes were in fact below 2,500, then lists in these southern regions would still not have risen above the criterion, though they would obviously have risen somewhat. This conclusion is of some importance. The key to the persistent manpower problems in parts of the midlands and the north may lie as much in seeking means of selective control over the outward flow of GPs as in the encouragement of more practitioners to move there. A successful long-term policy to dissuade young doctors who start out in the under-serviced regions from leaving for the attractions of the south would seem to stand a reasonable chance of easing the chronic shortage of family doctors in certain parts of the country.

The pattern of regional losses in Table A10 can be summarised by saying that doctors leaving each region have gone mainly to the South-East and to adjacent regions. Relative to size, however, it is only adjacent regions which are over-represented among the host regions, for the large numbers of doctors moving to the South-East merely reflects the fact that almost two-fifths of all principals in England live there. The pull of neighbouring regions is seen throughout the country. Most doctors moving out of the Northern region finished up in Yorkshire/Humberside and the North-West; those leaving Yorkshire went mainly to the North and the East Midlands;

those from the West Midlands were attracted to the East Midlands, the North-West and the South-West; and so on. The destinations of doctors moving out of the South-East showed a similar tendency to transfer to nearby regions. Three adjacent regions (the East and West Midlands and the South-West) accepted the highest absolute numbers, and relative to its size the East Anglian share was also large. In the North and in Yorkshire, by contrast, the numbers of GPs from the South-East were low, and the North-West also received a small proportion relative to its size.

The components of the balance of internal regional migration: gross gains

Since the analysis in this chapter deals with a closed system, the losses from one region are the gains to another. The picture of internal migration is therefore completed by considering the gross regional gains resulting from the movement of doctors within the country (columns 5 and 6 in Table A8). As with the losses, the gains vary considerably from region to region, but they differ somewhat from the expected pattern. Although the absolute number of doctors moving to the South-East has been large, this region, together with the South-West, the North and Yorkshire/Humberside, has gained the lowest proportion of doctors – about a fifth in each case. Then come the West Midlands and the North-West with slightly larger proportional gains, and finally the remaining two regions with appreciably higher gross percentage gains: East Anglia (32 per cent) and the East Midlands (52 per cent).

The conclusion drawn in the previous section concerning the relationship between the movement of doctors out of regions and the current regional distribution of manpower is to some extent strengthened by the lack of a corresponding relationship between a region's *attractiveness* to mobile doctors and its present stock of practitioners. The capacity to retain existing practitioners appears in this context to be more important than the ability to lure doctors from elsewhere. The East Midlands, for example, has attracted a very high proportion of doctors from other regions and yet still has a severe shortage, whilst the South-West, which has attracted a much lower proportion of GPs from elsewhere, has maintained a consistently low average list size.

The sources from which different regions have drawn their gross gains are a mirror-image of the losses (Table A10, reading down the columns). Just as most of the losses from each region were to the South-East and to neighbouring regions, so were most of the gains made from the South-East and from adjacent regions. The Northern region, as an example, made most of its gains from the South-East, from Yorkshire/Humberside and from the North-West; most of the doctors moving into Yorkshire in turn came from the North-West, the South-East and the East Midlands; and so on. The upshot of these reciprocal moves is that much of the total activity of internal mobility is self-cancelling: doctors moving from A to B have, over a period of time, more or less been replaced by equal numbers of GPs making the reverse trip. Hence the *net* balance of internal migration (that is, when all reciprocal moves are excluded) has generally revealed much smaller gains or losses to each region than the gross movements might suggest. In six of the eight regions, for example, the change through the net balance of internal migration has been less than or only a little above 10 per cent of those first practising there, and in the other two regions the change has been below 20 per cent. But even though the net changes to each region have been quite small, they are considerably larger than the net change either between the north and south of the country, or between the better-doctored and the under-doctored regions. After excluding reciprocal moves the *status quo* has virtually been preserved in the proportion of practitioners in the northern and the southern regions of the country, and in those with average list sizes above and below 2,500. The slight movement that has occurred has been in favour of the northern regions, but the net gain is of the order of less than one per cent. It may be seen as a hopeful indicator, but it is a very small one.

Inward migration from countries outside England

One further process completes the total picture of migration: the inflow of doctors to England from other countries.[3] Although the description of these people as 'immigrants' may suggest that they are foreign-born, this is not in fact the case. Most had been in general practice in other parts of the United Kingdom before moving to England: almost half had been in Scotland, a fifth in Wales, and a tenth in Northern Ireland. Only about 20 per cent of them had come from outside the UK, and fewer than one per cent of all the respondents in the survey had been born *and* had started in general practice outside the United Kingdom.

It is estimated that some 1,300 principals practising in England at the time of the survey had started their careers in general practice (either as assistants, trainees or principals) outside the country. The number is by no means insignificant for it roughly equals the total number of family doctors in the Northern or East Midland regions. Columns 9 and 10 in Table A8 show that, as a percentage of the number of doctors first practising in each region, these immigrants have been distributed fairly evenly throughout the country. The East Midlands and the North have attracted a higher than average proportion, and East Anglia has done rather less well than average, but there are no very large inter-regional differences in this respect. Even if they were optimally located, these immigrant doctors could not quite succeed in reducing the average list size in each region to 2,500, but they could go a long way towards doing so. For example, the 'excess' number in the three southern regions alone almost matched the total regional shortfall of GPs in 1970. Naturally this kind of numerical juggling depends upon an ideal distribution within each region which in reality could never be achieved, but the analysis illustrates the potential contribution which these doctors could make towards the problem of regional inequalities. They are a particularly important group because they are by definition highly mobile, and it is possible that with sufficient incentives they may be willing to move greater distances than doctors with stronger local ties.

Migration between counties

The regional migration analyses described in the previous sections can be repeated for each geographical county, and this has in fact been done as part of the full analysis of the survey data. The detailed figures are not presented here, however, partly because of space and partly because the small sample frequencies in some cases would make any conclusions relating to several individual counties highly tentative. Some broad observations about the inter-county migration patterns can nevertheless be made.

The most important conclusion is that even at the county level there has probably been sufficient potential in the observed migration patterns to ensure a currently equal distribution of doctors. The argument that certain counties have been basically unable to attract enough doctors to meet their current needs is difficult to sustain, for even allowing for the standard errors in the population estimates the gross losses of doctors from each county have been considerably in excess of the current shortfalls. As with the regions, the problem appears to be as much one of retaining GPs practising in certain areas as of enticing them there in the first place. This bald assertion, though fundamentally valid, must nevertheless be modified as a guide to pragmatic action. As in the regions, the relationship between past losses and present shortfalls is the outcome of long-term trends, for although the outflow of family doctors from each county has exceeded the current deficit, the total losses have built up over a long period of time. Even if the outward movement of GPs from certain counties could somehow be controlled it would still require several years before significant improvements in doctor/patient ratios were visible. At best, therefore, the implications of this analysis are long-term, and immediate improvements need to be sought through alternative channels. Further, the problem of retaining doctors in critical counties (and regions also) is primarily one of providing sufficient practice opportunities, for many of the doctors who had left an area would obviously not have gone there in the first place unless a vacancy had been created by the emigration of an existing practitioner. We return to this point later.

A second major conclusion from the study of inter-county migration is that, as with the regions, counties appear to differ in the extent to which their inability to retain doctors has contributed to their overall shortage. Some counties with very low rates of outward movement have still maintained quite large average lists, and although the shortage in these places could theoretically have been eliminated by reducing the losses still further, this would probably have been extremely difficult if not impossible to achieve. In these counties the most hopeful future developments are likely to come from increasing the intake of family doctors (from whatever source) rather than stemming the outward flow still further. There seems, moreover, to be an interesting north/south split in this respect. Counties in the northern regions have generally experienced a below-average loss of doctors moving elsewhere, and it is unlikely that the retention rate in these counties could be improved by any significant amount. Durham, Lancashire and the East and West Ridings are examples of northern counties which, despite a below-average loss, still experience large average lists. The particular problem in these counties seems to be the low capacity for attracting doctors moving from practices in other counties or immigrant doctors from outside England. In the South and the Midlands, on the other hand, the problem is more one of controlling losses than of stimulating gains, for although the under-doctored counties in these regions have generally experienced large gains of incoming doctors, they have also suffered high rates of outward movement of those first practising in them.

Mobility and manpower distribution

In this concluding section we attempt to draw some of the themes of the chapter together by relating the mobility patterns described so far to shortages in the distribution of general practitioners in 1969. (For technical reasons it has not been possible to carry out this particular exercise with 1970 data, but any changes during the year are probably quite small.) An area may be short of doctors either because it has attracted a lower-than-average proportion of those entering general practice for the first time, or because it has failed to get a fair share of practitioners moving from other areas or coming into the country from outside, or because it has lost an above-average number of doctors starting in that area but subsequently moving elsewhere. In this section we have calculated the effect on all the regions and counties in 1969 if each had achieved an average performance on each type of movement. The results are set out in Table A11. Regions and counties listed in the 'inadequate' column are those which, in spite of having an actual list size above 2,500 would, nevertheless, have been below this figure in 1969 if they had achieved an average performance on each growth factor *alone*. Conversely, those in the 'super-adequate' column would still have enjoyed average lists below 2,500 even if their performance on each factor alone had been no more than average. By concentrating on areas which would be thus affected by an average achievement on each *single* factor we can highlight the major strengths and weaknesses of the various regions and counties and also avoid the error of placing too much significance upon subtle changes revealed on the basis of rather small numbers. In practice, however, the situation in any region or county is obviously most likely to change as the result of partial improvement on several or all of the factors.

Table A11 shows how the flows of general practitioners through the country have affected list sizes from place to place. Results of this kind do not of themselves resolve the problem of under-doctored areas, but by contributing towards a clearer understanding of its nature and causes they should provide a better basis on which to build a policy. We hope this chapter has at least demonstrated the potential value of a systematic, continuous monitoring of the geographical movements of GPs, the results of which would be more valid than the limited analyses offered here. For however interesting our results may be, the data contain a number of imperfections. One is the inability to plot movements between sub-regional units with any confidence. Another is the problem of sorting out time trends in cross-sectional data, although separate checks on the migration patterns described in this chapter indicate that the major routes have probably changed little since 1948. For example, the regional distributions of the respondents' *first* and *current* appointments in general practice were very similar for those in different age groups, although it does not necessarily follow that the gross movements making up this net result must also be similar.

A more serious deficiency arises from the definition of 'losses' and 'gains' which were imposed upon us by the cross-sectional nature of the study. The conclusion in the preceding sections that the gross numbers of doctors moving out of each region and county has always exceeded the current shortfalls in those units may be questioned on the grounds that many of those moving out would only have moved *in* initially as replacements for other departing practitioners. It may therefore be considered misleading to regard the total number of doctors first practising in any unit as a cumulative statistic, implying that by retaining them all there would now be a sufficient stock of practitioners. The argument is a reasonable one, which could not be employed against longitudinal data collected from an on-going surveillance programme. Yet the fact remains that the total losses from each unit represent the gross number of doctors who were once practising there but are no longer doing so. The probability that they might not have gone in the first place unless another doctor had moved out does not invalidate the fact that they *did* still go, however undesirable or unattractive the place might be. There does not appear, therefore, to be any region or county that is *inherently* unable to attract enough family doctors to meet its needs (at least when needs are defined in terms of doctor/patient ratios) provided the practice opportunities are available.

7 The importance of community ties

> I should probably have settled in Edinburgh and gone into partnership with my uncle, but then I moved around and met my wife, and I finished up here. My father-in-law was in practice here.
>
> GP in Sussex

> I met a nice young lady here, so I stayed.
>
> GP in Leicestershire

Results of the kind presented in the previous chapter are important in reaching a clearer understanding of the nature of the problem of the designated areas, but they offer few clues about possible remedial action. It is instructive to know that the shortage of doctors in the East Midland counties is closely linked to the relatively low number of doctors first entering general practice who choose to go there, but this fact alone casts little light upon the steps which might effectively be taken to remedy the deficit. A rational course of action would first require some understanding of the reasons why younger doctors have been seemingly reluctant to enter general practice in the East Midlands. In the search for possible explanations this example of the East Midlands itself offers a clue, for it may be no coincidence that this was also the only region at the time of the survey without a medical school. (The medical faculty at Nottingham University did not accept its first students until 1970.) The absence of a medical school means that doctors in training have little opportunity of acquainting themselves with practice conditions within the region or of developing more general social contacts. The lack of such opportunity may later be important, for during his years at medical school the student will probably establish links with the local medical community and may build up an impression of practice conditions within the vicinity of the school which will subsequently be of some significance to him in evaluating possible areas of work. But at the same time other conflicting constraints may be operating on the student. He may be under some pressure to return to his family home area upon qualifying, especially if his father or some other relative is already practising there and has hopes of passing the practice on to the next generation. If he is married or engaged, then the further question of his wife's or fiancée's wishes and preferences may have to be incorporated into the decision of where to practise. In short, a strong relationship may exist between the places where GPs choose to work and the areas where they were born, grew up and were educated. It is with this relationship that this chapter is concerned.

Previous research

It seems often to have been assumed that doctors (especially general practitioners) tend to settle in the vicinity of their medical schools, and that consequently the careful siting of new medical schools and the expansion of existing ones would offer a reasonable long-term solution to recruitment problems in certain areas. If, the argument runs, there is an increase in the number of students who are trained in a particular locality, there will also be an increase in the number who choose to settle there upon qualifying.[1] The Gillie Report in 1963, for instance, commented that 'since there is a tendency for doctors to enter general practice in the part of the country in which they were trained, new medical schools and medical centres for post-graduate training should, as far as possible, be in or close to the under-doctored areas'.[2] The argument was repeated in the following year by the Working Party on General Practice.[3] 'Doctors tend to settle in the areas in which they were trained and we think it important that the uneven distribution of general practitioners should be borne in mind when considering the location of new medical schools and the expansion of existing ones.' Neither report cited any evidence for the argument, although both committees would have had access to the Medical Practices Committee's analysis of the Provisional Register for 1960, indicating that doctors normally settled in and about the areas where they had been educated.[4] Probably the first major survey of the settlement patterns of doctors was published in 1967 by Last.[5] His results certainly confirmed the widespread belief that medical schools tend to supply GPs to adjacent rather than to remoter regions, but he also found that a closer association existed between the places where GPs worked and the areas of their family homes at the time they were students. In fact, just over half (51 per cent) of all the general practitioners in his nationwide sample were practising in the same standard region as their family home. Last concluded that 'regions short of doctors would be more effectively, expediently and economically helped to overcome the shortage by a larger recruitment of students from these regions, rather than by establishing medical schools there'.

The Royal Commission on Medical Education,[6] echoing Last's conclusion, commented that 'the argument about settlement introduces unnecessary and misleading considerations' into decisions about the siting of new medical schools. The Commission pointed out that although some of the plans which had been submitted to it about the location of new schools were based on the assumption that medical graduates tended to practise in the area of their medical schools, there was in fact no substantial evidence to support it. Last's material was used to show that the evidence which did exist pointed the other way, and indicated that general practitioners, if not consultants, preferred to return to their home areas to work. However, the Commission did think that the supply of general practitioners to an area 'may well be heavily dependent on the extent to which boys and girls from that area are attracted into medicine', and that one way of attracting them may be to set up a local medical school. It would appear, then, that both home area and medical school are likely to be significant factors in the choice of a practice location, but whether they act independently of each other has yet to be established.

The more intensive studies by Brown and Walker in East Yorkshire, Glamorgan and South Hampshire confirm this conclusion.[7,8] They found that 41 per cent of the 260 doctors interviewed in these three localities had parents living in the same region (the comparable figure from Last's national survey was 51 per cent, although definitions do not exactly match), and 24 per cent had parents in the same town or village. Younger doctors were more likely to have returned to their home areas than those graduating before the war, and the Welsh doctors had closer connections than those in either of the English regions. Moreover, 68 per cent of all GPs in the sample were in the area of their first choice. At the same time, however, the results showed that the medical school also represented a considerable constraint on the range of a doctor's choice: by 1966 a third of the general practitioners in the East and West Ridings were Leeds graduates, and in Glamorgan the proportion of graduates from the Welsh National School of Medicine was 50 per cent. Brown and Walker concluded that 'recruitment of general practitioners is likely to be easiest in areas that send substantial numbers of schoolboys and girls to medical school. . . . We cannot dismiss the need to bear this factor in mind in siting new medical schools.'

The influence of community ties: the national picture

This section examines the relationship between home area, medical school and practice location. (Family home area is defined by the question: 'Where did you spend most of your time before going to University?') In the designated sample almost two-fifths (39 per cent) of respondents whose family homes had been in England were practising in the same *county* as their family home, and 60 per cent were practising in the same standard *region.* The corresponding proportions in the non-designated sample were 37 per cent and 60 per cent. (It is important to note that these figures apply only to respondents whose family homes had been in England. Since the survey was restricted to GPs in England it would clearly have been misleading to include *all* respondents in this analysis as they would not have been at equal risk of being counted in their home localities.) The regional figures correspond well with the equivalent proportion in Last's survey (51 per cent), even though his definition of family home differed somewhat from ours, and they indicate the substantial attraction which a doctor's home area has for him in later life. But a similar attraction is exerted by the medical school, for almost identical proportions of respondents were, at the time of the survey, practising in the counties and regions of the teaching hospitals at which they trained as undergraduates. In the designated sample 32 per cent of those trained in England were currently practising in the same *county* and 60 per cent in the same *region* as their medical school, and the corresponding proportions in the non-designated sample were 27 per cent and 54 per cent.

It therefore follows that many of the doctors must have trained not far from their homes, and the question arises of whether the attraction of each is independent of the other. If the influence of the medical school is independent of the home area then the proportion of respondents practising in the vicinity of their schools would be no different as between those whose family homes had and had not also been in the same region as their medical schools. In fact the results show that this is not the case, for the chances of a doctor remaining in the region of his medical school were much higher if that had also been his family home region. For example, the proportions of doctors in the designated sample practising in the same region as their medical school varied from 70 per cent among those trained in their home region to only 29 per cent among those trained elsewhere. In the non-designated sample the corresponding figures were 65 per cent and 29 per cent, showing an equally wide range. (In both samples the percentages are based upon the number of respondents whose family homes *and* medical schools had been in England. The reasons for this have already been given.) Similar results were to be seen at the county level also. The proportion of designated doctors practising in the same county as their medical school ranged from 48 per cent among those trained in their home county to only 16 per cent among those trained elsewhere, and the corresponding figures in the non-designated sample were 46 per cent and 12 per cent.

These results demonstrate unequivocally that although the majority of GPs graduating from English universities settle within the regional vicinity of their universities, the attraction of the medical school is much greater when it also happens to be located in the region of the family home. But the converse question, hitherto unanswered in previous studies, is whether it is not equally the case that doctors are more likely to settle in the vicinity of their family home if that also happens to be where they were trained. The answer is again in the affirmative. The proportion of designated doctors working in the same standard regions as their family homes varied from 70 per cent of those trained in their home regions to only 32 per cent of those who left their home regions to go to medical school. Similarly, the proportions of non-designated doctors working in their home regions were 65 per cent and 48 per cent respectively as between those who were and were not also educated in their home regions. As before, the same trends applied also at the county level. In short, students who had left their home regions and counties to be trained were less likely to have returned to them as GPs than those attending a medical school in their home regions and counties. The general hypothesis which emerges may be stated thus: the more connections a doctor has with an area the more likely he is to return to it or remain in it to practise. If the hypothesis is valid we should expect to find the proportion of doctors living in their home areas to increase still further if, as well as being educated there, they were also born in those places. The upshot of incorporating birthplace into the analysis is that although its influence on practice location is considerably less than either home area or medical school, it nevertheless increases the likelihood that a GP will return to or remain in a familiar area by adding one more link to the chain which keeps him. The significance of each of these links is summarised in Table A12, which shows the proportions of respondents living in the same *regions* as their birthplace, home area and medical school under the various possible combinations.

Two major conclusions are drawn from this table. First, the proportion of GPs practising in any region increased in regular fashion as the total number of links with the region accumulated. In each case the proportion was lowest among doctors with just one link (whether that link was of birth, upbringing or education), and highest among those with all three links. Thus of doctors whose only link with a region was through their birthplace fewer than one in ten (8 per cent) were currently practising in that region. When one extra link is added (whether home or medical school) the proportion rises to at least 40 per cent, and when all three links are present more than two-thirds (67 per cent) of the respondents are accounted for.

The second principal conclusion suggested by Table A12 is that each link has a differential effect upon the probability of a doctor practising in the region in question. The influence of birthplace appears to be the slightest, for it has the lowest retention rate in isolation and the least incremental effect when added to either of the other two. By similar reasoning the home area has the strongest pull, with the medical school occupying an intermediate position. Schematically the relative influence of each link is illustrated in Diagram 2, adding for this purpose the extra link of the spouse's family home area which is discussed in greater detail in Chapter 8.

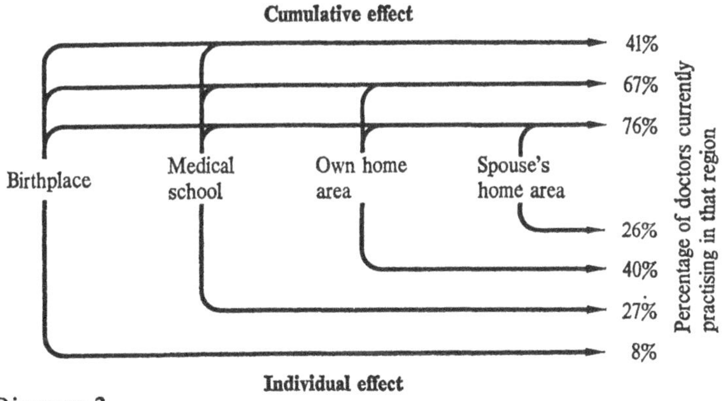

Diagram 2
(*Note* Percentages are based on weighted aggregates of both samples)

This analysis of the relationship between home area, location of medical school and choice of practice area adds a further dimension to the results of previous studies. Our results confirm the importance of encouraging more young people in under-doctored areas to consider medicine as a career, because wherever they are trained at least a third of them can be expected to return to their home regions. But it has also been shown that this proportion is likely to double if students can receive their medical education in their home regions, and that is the rationale for locating new medical schools and expanding existing ones in such areas. Our results support Last's conclusion that the influence of the home is greater than that of the university, but we cannot accept the Royal Commission's argument about the irrelevance of the siting of medical schools to manpower policy. This survey has clearly shown that the influence of the home area and the medical school are interdependent, and the effects of both should be considered equally.

The influence of community ties: the regional and county picture

The conclusions in the previous section were pitched at the level of the country as a whole: the next step is to examine their validity in relation to each region and county. If the conclusion is valid that doctors who attend medical schools in their home regions are more likely to be practising in those regions than doctors who move away for their training, then we should expect to find that those regions in which a high proportion of students had trained 'at home' would also have the highest rates of retention of home-bred doctors. The figures are set out in Table A13, and are confined to respondents whose family homes had been in England. The first column shows, for each region, the percentage of respondents who had been to a medical school in the same region as their family home. The South-East expectedly had the highest proportion of doctors training in their home region (88 per cent); the North, Yorkshire/Humberside, the North-West and the West Midlands each had between 60 and 70 per cent; and in the South-West the proportion was 27 per cent. No doctors with family homes in the East Midlands had received their medical education there, and the very low proportion in East Anglia is due to the fact that, wherever possible, Cambridge graduates were classified by the location of their clinical school. These regional variations partly reflect the capacity of the medical schools, but it would nevertheless be possible in principle for a higher proportion of students to be trained in their home regions than has hitherto been the case, for between a fifth and a third of undergraduate places in each region usually go to students originating from other regions. Since the chances of a GP practising in his family home area increase if he also attends a medical school nearby, this might be a possible way of using existing resources to encourage more GPs to settle in selected regions.

Next, we should expect to find that regions which trained a high proportion of indigenous students would also contain a high proportion of GPs practising in their home regions. The figures in the second column of Table A13 show that the retention rate was indeed highest in the South-East, where 65 per cent of doctors with family homes in the region were still practising, and lowest (by a considerable margin) in the East Midlands (39 per cent). Between these extremes the other regions ranged much as expected, although in most cases the rank positions are admittedly determined by quite small percentage variations. The major exception is the South-Western region, which despite losing a very high proportion of students to other regions to be trained has nevertheless succeeded in attracting back a large number of those originating from the region.

The results of the analysis at county level are much more speculative, partly because of the small sample frequencies in several cases and partly because very few counties actually contain medical schools. The best results are those relating to the proportion of doctors with family homes in each county who had, at the time of the survey, returned to them as GPs. Counties in the South-East generally had low proportions. Only Hampshire among these counties had a retention rate above the average for all counties (37 per cent), whilst no more than one in ten of those with family homes in Oxfordshire, Bedfordshire and Buckinghamshire had returned to these counties. Counties in the Northern region, by contrast, have had much more success, for all except the North Riding have managed to retain at least half the doctors with family homes in them. In Yorkshire/Humberside, the East and West Ridings together have kept a higher proportion of home-produced doctors (57 per cent) than any other county except Cornwall, contrasting dramatically with the low figure of 16 per cent in the North Riding. All the constituent counties in the East Midlands have followed the regional trend of retaining a fairly low proportion of doctors with family homes in them, whilst those in East Anglia have succeeded in keeping at least the national average proportion. So also have Devon, Cornwall and Dorset in the South-West, although the remaining three counties in this region have done less well. The larger counties in the West Midlands have had difficulty in retaining reasonable numbers of doctors with family homes in them: the proportion was only a third in Warwickshire and Staffordshire and no more than a quarter in Worcestershire. Finally, in the North-West, Lancashire has retained proportionately twice as many home-bred doctors as Cheshire, which is doubtless due in part to the presence of two medical schools in Lancashire.

The relationship between attendance at a local medical school and the probability of practising in the vicinity of the family home is obviously much less clear at county than at regional level. Nevertheless with the exception of those counties from which fewer than ten of the survey doctors had originated, most counties with medical schools had a higher proportion of home-bred doctors than those without. It seems safe to conclude that the presence of a local medical school usually ensures that a good proportion of medical students from the area will eventually return as GPs.

The influence of community ties: the relationship to the distribution of manpower

The next crucial question is whether the trends described in the preceding sections have affected the distribution of family doctors. Has the failure of certain regions and counties to retain an adequate proportion of home-based doctors been a significant factor in the manpower shortage in those areas? The results discussed above suggest that a link may exist at both regional and county level between the capacity to retain home-bred doctors and the current availability of manpower. The link is revealed most explicitly in the East Midlands and North-West, which not only stand out by virtue of the relatively low numbers of indigenous doctors taking a first appointment in them (the third column in Table A13), but are also the two regions in which a low capacity to attract doctors entering general practice has been a major reason underlying their current shortages (Table A11). The younger doctors whom these regions have failed to attract may, in other words, be those whose family homes were in the regions but who took a first appointment elsewhere. If both regions had retained merely an average proportion of GPs taking a first appointment in their home regions the extra doctors gained would have offset the 1970 deficits completely. Moreover the situation in the East Midlands is a clear example of how recruiting problems can be intensified by the lack of a medical teaching centre, and it is expected that the opening of the medical school at Nottingham will exert a significant long-term influence on staffing patterns in the region.

A similar conclusion can be drawn from the county data. Eleven counties were listed in Table A11 in which the failure to attract enough doctors entering general practice has been a principal reason underlying their current shortage of GPs. In each of these eleven counties the proportion of doctors taking a first appointment in their home counties was lower than average, with the exception of Durham/Northumberland and Lancashire (which contain medical schools) and Huntingdonshire (which has only two cases and can therefore be disregarded). What does this imply? Having shown that the shortage of doctors in many counties has resulted mainly from the failure to attract into general practice, the problem can now be located more specifically in the low proportions of doctors originating from those counties who have returned to them as GPs. Whilst it is impossible to base any firm conclusions on a small number of cases it is probably no coincidence that the two counties in this group containing medical schools have generally shown much higher retention rates than those without an undergraduate medical centre. It seems clear from all the evidence that a medical school which a doctor attends is likely to be an important influence in his choice of a practice area, and that in some cases it may be a contributory factor in the maldistribution of GPs. These results are quite contrary in their implication to the assertion of the Todd Commission that the siting of new medical schools is irrelevant to the problems of manpower distribution. Our data indicate very clearly that a promising way of bolstering recruitment to general practice in many under-doctored areas is by encouraging more doctors originating from those areas to return to them when qualified, and further, that one way of promoting this is to ensure that they do not have to travel far from home in order to be trained.

Which doctors return home?

Which doctors are most likely to return to their home areas as GPs? Table A14 sets out some characteristics *of those respondents with family homes in England* who at the time of the survey were living in the same county and region as their family home. Three of the characteristics discriminate decisively between those who had returned home and those who had not. The first concerns the timing of a doctor's marriage relative to his career in general practice: respondents in both samples who had married before entering general practice were rather more likely than the remainder to be working away from their home regions and counties. The spouse's influence, discussed in the next chapter, may be a factor here. The second discriminating characteristic is paternal occupation. Respondents were asked to record their fathers' occupations at the time they (the respondents) were born, and these were then classified on the Registrar-General's social class scale, and also according to their relationship with medicine. Those whose fathers had also been doctors were more likely to be practising in their home counties than those with fathers in other occupations, and were less likely to be practising in a different region. The difference is consistent in both samples, but most marked in the non-designated sample. Associated with this is the fact that doctors originating from social class I homes contained relatively more of those returning to their home counties and regions than respondents with fathers in other social classes. The many important contacts which a newly qualified doctor may have in his home area by virtue of his father's practice is probably sufficient explanation for his increased incentive to return, especially if there is the prospect of a partnership in the family practice.

The influence of age is more difficult to assess because the younger doctors in the survey had not yet completed all their career moves. A correct interpretation of the slight trend (more marked in the designated than the non-designated sample) towards a higher rate of settlement in home regions by younger doctors is therefore a hazardous matter, but it seems possible that they may be genuinely more likely than their older colleagues to remain within the regional vicinity of their family homes throughout their careers, even though they may change practices more often.

The capacity of medical schools and the supply of medical students

In this concluding section we explore the possibility that some regions may fail to produce enough students in the first place because of the lack of undergraduate places. The question of whether or not the local availability of such places stimulates the number of qualified school leavers who choose to study medicine was considered by the Royal Commission on Medical Education in 1968.[9] The survey of medical students carried out on behalf of the Commission in 1966 showed that in 1964–5 the number of undergraduate medical students as a proportion of *all* full-time university undergraduates ranged from 13·6 per cent in the South-East to zero in the East Midlands, with the remaining six regions ranged between 5·0 per cent in East Anglia[10] and 7·7 per cent in the West Midlands. On the other side of the equation, the number of entrants to medical school in that year (as a rate per 1,000 leavers with two or more 'A' levels in each region) varied from 16·2 in East Anglia to 31·1 in the West Midlands. The rank correlation on the two scores is moderately low (rho = 0·40), but it did emerge from the 1966 survey that the two regions without a clinical school (i.e. the East Midlands and East Anglia) had a relatively poor record of supplying entrants to the medical school. After allowing for the degree of encouragement which teachers in different regions gave to school-leavers aiming at a medical career, and the social class structure of the populations, the survey authors concluded that 'East Anglia and to a lesser extent the East Midlands are contributing less to medical education than the other regions and could contribute more than they do now'. It is instructive to note that the East Midland region is thus consistently deficient on each measure: its school-leavers receive the least encouragement from teachers to study medicine, it produces fewer medical students than most other regions, it retains the lowest proportion taking up their first appointments in general practice, and it has the lowest proportion of home-produced doctors currently working in the region. When all of these facts are set against the extra one that the East Midlands had no medical school at all when these figures were compiled, then the potential significance of the location of undergraduate medical teaching centres is highlighted dramatically.

8 The doctor as a person

> My ancestors have been practising medicine in an almost unbroken line in this area since 1680.
>
> GP in Northumberland

The analysis of the survey data in the previous three chapters placed heavy emphasis on biographical and career features. We have attempted to show how the doctors in the survey had changed practices and moved from one location to another during the course of their careers, and to evaluate the significance of the historical attachments of birth, upbringing and education in the choice of practice location. The remainder of the analysis is concerned more with the present, and seeks to establish the differences, if any, between practices and practitioners in different parts of the country and in different types of practice areas. The purpose is two-fold: first, to provide a descriptive outline of the state of general practice in different geographical locations, and second, to elaborate the factors which might predispose doctors to choose certain localities or types of area in which to live. This chapter is concerned with the personal attributes of age, sex, social class, marriage and family responsibilities.

Age

The age distributions of respondents in different types of practice areas were very similar. Those in designated areas were slightly younger than their colleagues elsewhere, but the differences were not large. The median age of doctors in designated areas was 45·7 years, compared with 47·6, 46·8 and 48·3 years respectively in open, intermediate and restricted areas. At the extremes of the age range there were slightly more younger doctors and fewer older doctors in designated than in non-designated areas, suggesting that the decline in manpower resulting from retirement during the next ten years or so may be felt most sharply in those areas which at present enjoy a relative superfluity of practitioners. Against this, if figures were available of the average age of retirement in each practice area they might show that GPs in designated areas retired younger than those elsewhere. Such evidence would account for the slightly lower proportion of older GPs in these areas without endorsing our forecast of lower retirement rates there during the next decade. But for the time being our results cast doubt upon the evidence submitted to and accepted by the Review Body in 1970 that the chronically under-doctored areas carry the greatest risks of retirement and death resulting in a serious dislocation of services.[1]

The age distributions of GPs in each standard region were also similar. Indeed, less than two years separated the lowest and highest regional median ages – the East Midlands (45·6) and the South-East and South-West (47·3). Regional disparities were slightly more marked at the extremes of the age range. Only the two midland regions had more than a quarter of GPs under the age of 40 (in most regions the proportion was about a fifth), whilst East Anglia, with fewer than 10 per cent of principals over the age of 60, will probably suffer less from the future effects of retirement than most other regions. These differences, however, are largely ones of detail, and do not substantially modify the overwhelming impression that, at least in terms of their age, doctors in different practice areas and standard regions were very similar people.

Sex

About 10 per cent of all principals in England and Wales are women, a sufficiently low proportion to make them a seemingly insignificant factor in the problem of manpower distribution, but one which, nevertheless, represents quite a large absolute number of practitioners (2,158 unrestricted principals in 1971). Since the number of women doctors in full-time work (though not necessarily in general practice) amounts to no more than half of all those qualified, the question arises of whether a low rate of employment among women GPs is at least a contributory factor in the overall shortage of medical personnel in certain areas. The evidence from previous surveys suggests a negative answer, for the proportion of medically qualified women in full-time work is generally higher in large urban areas where opportunities are relatively plentiful than in more sparsely populated rural stretches.[2,3]

The present survey can show neither the total number of qualified women resident in each area nor the proportion employed in general practice, but it can show the proportion of women among the respondents from each area. Failure to make the fullest possible use of women doctors might be suspected as a factor in the shortage of GPs in designated areas if they were shown to constitute a lower proportion there than in non-designated areas. This is in fact the case, for whereas women doctors constituted one in ten of all the non-designated sample, they accounted for only 6 per cent of the designated sample. The difference, however, is insufficiently large to be considered a realistic factor in the shortage of doctors. Variations between the regions were much greater. The proportion of women respondents was considerably lower in the South-East and South-West than in the rest of the country, and was high in East Anglia, the North-West and, to a lesser degree, in the two midland regions. There is no clear relationship between the proportion of women doctors in a region and the regional average list size, but if it is assumed that the number of qualified women at risk of being recruited into general practice is approximately the same in each region (relative to size) then it follows that some regions may not have fully exploited this additional resource. It is extremely unlikely that the designated areas could be entirely eliminated in this way, even if all non-employed women doctors were recruited immediately to general practice, but this extra source of 'manpower' could probably make a significant improvement in many local areas.

Social class and educational background

The classification of doctors in each area by the social class of their family of origin reveals a number of interesting points (Table A15). Most striking is the very large proportion of respondents in each area from social class I (i.e. professional) backgrounds. In total, 32 per cent of the designated sample and 40 per cent of the non-designated sample had fathers in professional occupations, and this grossly exceeds the figure for the general adult population.[4] Conversely, a very low proportion of respondents had fathers in semi-skilled or unskilled manual occupations (3 per cent and 1 per cent respectively). Other studies of the medical profession confirm this finding, both in the United States and in this country. In America, more than half the medical students graduating in 1960 had fathers who were professionals, proprietors or managers,[5] although there is some evidence of an increasing 'democratization of recruitment' to the profession throughout the first half of the century.[6] In this country, Brown and Walker found that 43 per cent of their sample of GPs in East Yorkshire, Hampshire and Glamorgan had fathers in class I occupations,[7] and, as the Todd Commission pointed out, the proportion of doctors drawn from the higher social classes is increasing. The 1966 survey of medical students carried out for the Commission showed that 34 per cent of all final-year students in 1961 and 1966 came from social class I homes, and among first-year students in 1966 the proportion was 40 per cent.[8] Comparison with the general student population is difficult, but the Robbins Report on Higher Education[9] showed that 59 per cent of a sample of undergraduates in 1961 came from class I and II backgrounds, compared with the figure of 73 per cent among medical students in the ASME survey in the same year.

The chances of becoming a doctor are therefore many times greater for a child from a professional than from a working-class background, and this is wholly consistent with the large volume of evidence that children from middle-class homes are much more likely to achieve educational success than those from poorer backgrounds, even when intellectual ability is taken into account.[10] In the case of doctors, however, there is the added factor of 'self-recruitment' – that is, of children following in their fathers' occupational footsteps.[11] Almost a quarter (23 per cent) of the GPs in our survey were themselves the children of doctors, an identical proportion to that found by Brown and Walker and a similar one to that among final-year medical students in 1966 (21 per cent).[12,13] Self-recruitment is generally higher in medicine than in other professions.[14] The tendency for the children of doctors to choose a medical career themselves is doubtless due in part to the natural processes of anticipatory socialisation within the medical family.[15] Medically qualified parents possess the means and the motives for generating and nurturing medical ambitions in their children; as Hall puts it, 'only the members of a profession can translate the public protestations of the profession into the vernacular of useful advice'.[16] But this type of explanation, applicable to any profession, would not explain the exceptionally high degree of self-recruitment in medicine. The rest of the explanation may lie in the greater visibility of medical work (especially general practice) to the children of doctors, and also in the selection procedures adopted by the medical schools which may be weighted in favour of applicants from medical families.

Although the doctors in the survey were, as a whole, drawn from high-class backgrounds, there were nevertheless some consistent differences between those in each type of practice area. Just under a third of respondents in designated areas had fathers in class I jobs, with the percentage rising through the open and intermediate areas to a peak of 47 per cent among those in restricted areas. Against this, the other non-manual classes (II and III non-manual) were slightly over-represented in the designated sample, though not sufficiently to counter-balance the trend in class I. Thus on a simple manual/non-manual dichotomy there were slightly fewer doctors from non-manual backgrounds in designated areas (81 per cent) than elsewhere, with those in restricted areas having the highest proportion (87 per cent). The relatively low proportion of designated doctors with fathers in social class I occupations is partly (though not entirely) explained by the fact that, compared with the others, fewer were themselves the children of doctors. Exactly a fifth of the designated doctors came from medical backgrounds, with the proportion rising to 30 per cent and 27 per cent respectively among those in intermediate and restricted areas.

Paralleling these social differences are variations in educational background. More doctors in the designated than in the non-designated sample had attended a grammar school (50 per cent against 40 per cent) and correspondingly fewer had been to a public school (39 per cent against 48 per cent). But even among doctors from class I backgrounds the designated sample contained fewer former public school pupils (59 per cent) than the non-designated sample (65 per cent). These differences accord very closely with the results of the 1966 ASME survey, and they are consistent with our earlier finding about the differential class structures of the two samples. It is, however, less significant and less surprising that the relationship between paternal social class and educational background holds good *within* each sample than that these considerable social differences should exist at all *between* doctors in different practice areas. Can they be explained in geographical terms; that is, do they disappear when geographical location is controlled? The answer is negative, at least at the regional level, for even *within* every region proportionately fewer designated than non-designated doctors had fathers in professional or managerial jobs, and more came from working-class homes. In some regions the differences were quite small, but their consistency sustains the conclusion that real differences in social class background existed between GPs in different types of practice areas which cannot be explained by regional factors.

Having made that point, however, some regional variations were nevertheless apparent in the class backgrounds of the respondents, for in both samples the three regions to the south of a line from the Wash to the Severn contained more doctors from middle-class origins than the midland and northern regions. These results can perhaps be explained by certain generalised features of family development. If it is assumed that higher-status people usually live in 'nicer' areas (which might crudely be equated with the non-designated areas), and that a substantial number of doctors return to their home areas to practise, this would account for the higher proportion of doctors from class I backgrounds in restricted than in designated areas. The relatively high preponderance of medically qualified parents among the former group would further accentuate the tendency. By contrast, doctors from poorer backgrounds, also tending to return to their home areas as qualified practitioners, would be rather more likely to finish up in a designated area, even though many of them will doubtless reside in a 'better' locality than their parents.

Marriage

Career decisions, particularly those involving movement from one place to another, may be influenced heavily by the obligations and restraints resulting from family responsibilities at different stages of the family cycle. It has already been seen how far these responsibilities and commitments may curtail the mobility potential of young doctors in general practice, for the timing of a doctor's marriage and the ages of his children appear to affect his chances of moving (Chapter 5). In the light of these findings it seems reasonable to ask whether such considerations might also affect decisions about where to live. For example, the lack of adequate educational facilities is part of the folklore of the designated areas and it might therefore be expected that doctors working in such places would be less likely than the rest to have been faced with imminent problems of education at the time they accepted their current appointments.[17] It is possible that fewer were married at the time or fewer had children. Spouses, too, are likely to have had an important influence on the decision. (Although the word 'spouse' is used for reasons of accuracy, most of them were in fact the wives of male doctors. About 8 per cent of the spouses were the husbands of female respondents.) The finding in the previous chapter that doctors who had married before entering general practice or before taking up their current appointments were more likely than the rest to be working away from their home regions and counties suggests that a spouse's preferences may modify or even compete with those of the doctor.

More than nine out of every ten doctors in each type of practice area and each standard region were married, approximately 4 per cent were single, 2 per cent widowed, and 1 per cent divorced or separated. The regional and area differences were not significant, nor were there any substantial variations in the time at which respondents had married relative to their entry into general practice. In each type of practice area about two-thirds had married before starting their careers in general practice and about a further 12 per cent had married after becoming GPs but before moving to their current appointments (Table A16). The remaining doctors had thus married *after* starting their present jobs, and this proportion is identical in both the designated and the non-designated samples (15 per cent). There is no support in these figures for the hypothesis that either the fact of being married or the timing of the marriage distinguishes doctors in the different types of practice areas.

The regional distribution of the spouses' home areas was very similar to that of the doctors themselves. (Spouse's home area is defined by the question: 'Where was your wife's (husband's) home for most of the time before her (his) marriage?' About a third of the spouses whose family homes had been in England were, at the time of the survey, living in the same *county* as their home and a further fifth were living in a different county of the same *region*. Put another way, just over half of all the doctors whose spouses had family homes in England were practising in the same standard region as their *spouses*' homes – slightly fewer than were working in the same region as their *own* family homes. There were no significant differences between the designated and non-designated samples in this respect. The conclusion from this finding, that the influence of the spouse's home area is closely tied up with that of the doctor's own home territory, is confirmed by the fact that 46 per cent of the designated sample and 43 per cent of the non-designated sample had married someone from their own home regions. The interesting question is whether the two influences operate independently. Are doctors more likely to be practising in their home regions if these are also the places of their spouses' family home? The answer is in the affirmative. Whereas 60 per cent of the designated doctors were living in the same standard region as their family home, the proportion increased to 75 per cent among those whose spouses also came from the region, and fell to 42 per cent for those who had married partners from a different region. Similarly, whereas 60 per cent of respondents in the non-designated sample were practising in their home region, the proportions were 72 per cent and 42 per cent respectively for those whose spouses did and did not have their family homes in the same regions. The differences also held good at the county level. (For reasons discussed in the previous chapter these figures are limited to respondents whose own *and* spouses' family homes had been in England.)

The *independent* influence of the spouse's home area (that is, when it is unrelated to the doctor's birthplace, own home area or medical school) seems to rank on a par with the medical school: more significant than a doctor's birthplace but less so than his own home area. Thus 26 per cent of respondents for whom all the relevant geographical points were in England were currently practising in the same standard region as their spouses' homes when they had none of the other recorded links with it, and there were no differences in this respect between the two samples. Where the spouse's home added an extra link to the chain of association which a doctor had with a region, then the chances of his living there increased still further. Whereas some two-thirds of the doctors who were born, brought up and medically educated in the same region of England were also practising in that region, the figure rose to 76 per cent among those who had also married someone from the region (see Diagram 2).

Family responsibilities

The evidence from the survey about the relationship between family responsibilities, mobility, and choice of practice area shows an interesting divergence. On the one hand it is clear that in several ways the respondents' family commitments had limited the amount of movement which they made. The earlier they had married the less likely they were to have moved at all, and almost all had settled by the time their children reached secondary school age. On the other hand there is very little evidence that these factors had also affected decisions of *where* to practise, whether this is defined in the broad sense of the type of practice area, or in the more limited sense of the region of the country. One might expect the obvious and justified concern which doctors have about the education of their children to be reflected in their choice of a place to work, but this does not appear to be the case, at least in terms of the choice between a designated and a non-designated area (Table A17). Respondents in designated areas were no more likely than the rest to have started their current positions before having any children, and they were just as likely to have started by the time their eldest child had reached secondary school age. Part of the explanation may lie in the use made of boarding schools, about which we have no information. It may also mean that the perceived educational facilities of the area were unimportant to most respondents in accepting their current positions, although again we cannot be sure. But certainly for many doctors the problems of secondary education were fairly distant at the time they settled down, and they were as distant for those moving into what are now the non-designated areas as for the rest.

9 The doctor as a professional

> The government is already getting doctoring on the cheap in designated areas, and the strain is so great that an added inducement is needed to encourage more help. The appalling strain on a good doctor of not having time to take a proper history, or do thorough examinations, is never mentioned – but it is *his* conscience which suffers when there is a disaster, not the politicians.
>
> GP in London

Qualifications and medical school

The respondents in the survey held similar primary and secondary qualifications, whichever region or whatever type of practice area they were in. The proportion of doctors holding *only* an M.B., Ch.B. (or equivalent) fell consistently from 66 per cent of doctors in designated areas to 56 per cent of those in restricted areas, but this was offset by a compensating increase in the proportion of those holding an M.B., Ch.B. *and* conjoint (Table A18). Most of the medical schools from which these primary qualifications had been obtained were equally represented among doctors in each sample, with the exception of London University, which supplied 43 per cent of the doctors in the non-designated areas but only 28 per cent of those in designated areas. These figures probably reflect the position of London in relation to the geographical dispersion of designated areas rather than a deliberate bias against such areas on the part of London graduates. Graduates from medical schools outside England, and from the Royal Colleges, were fairly equally represented in each sample, and there is no consistent evidence that these doctors had been particularly biased towards or against certain types of practice areas. Doctors from Indian and Pakistani medical schools made up no more than 1·5 per cent of the total number of GPs in the survey, and, given the small numbers involved, were equally represented in the designated and non-designated samples.

This latter figure is instructive for the light it casts on the emotive question of foreign-born doctors in the National Health Service. The

1968 Annual Report of the Department of Health and Social Security showed that 13 per cent of all the unrestricted principals in England that year were born outside the British Isles, and the present survey for the same year yielded proportions of 11 per cent and 12 per cent respectively in the designated and non-designated samples. But the data also showed that the majority of these doctors had been born in non-Commonwealth countries; indeed, fewer than 5 per cent of all respondents had been born in Commonwealth countries, and even this figure over-estimates the proportion of Commonwealth citizens because birthplace does not necessarily define nationality. Many doctors who had been born in India, for example, were the sons of English parents on colonial service. A better estimate of the proportion of *Asian* doctors in general practice might be made on the basis of medical school attendance, and on this indicator the maximum proportion would be set at about 2–3 per cent. At the same time, however, the proportion of Asian GPs may well be increasing. Cargill's analysis of a 10 per cent sample of all practitioners in England and Wales showed that the proportion of graduates from Asian medical schools *entering* general practice increased from 4 per cent in 1961–2 to 18 per cent in 1969.[1] These figures are consistent with the conclusion that about 2-3 per cent of all principals *currently* in practice are of Asian origin, but it seems likely that this proportion is now rising.[2]

Age at starting current position

Although respondents in different practice areas and regions of the country had spent similar lengths of time in general practice and in their current positions, those in the designated sample had started their present positions at a slightly younger age than their colleagues elsewhere (Table A19). Whereas, for example, 42 per cent of all GPs in the designated sample had started in their current positions by the age of 30, only 37 per cent of the others had done so. The overall difference is admittedly small, but because it holds good in every age group between 34 and 55 it is probably a genuine difference rather than a mere quirk of the data. Moreover, the proportion of doctors in the 50–54 age group starting their present positions by the age of 30 was artificially low in both samples as a result of the disruptive effects of the war. It seems, therefore, that in areas which were designated at the time of the survey, it has usually been possible to become a principal at a slightly younger age than in the other areas, and this is as true for those who had made several moves as for those who had made none. Naturally the more moves a doctor had made the older he was, on average, when he started his current position, but even among those who had been in more than one practice there remained a higher proportion of designated than non-designated doctors starting in their present positions by the age of 30.

Other current appointments

The doctors in the survey were asked whether, in addition to their responsibilities in general practice, they held any other medical appointments. The proportion responding positively ranged from 56 per cent in designated areas to 66 per cent in restricted areas (Table A20). There were also some regional differences. A comparatively high proportion of doctors in the Northern region reported at least one other appointment, and the proportions were also quite high in the West Midlands, the South-East and South-West, and the Yorkshire/Humberside region. Conversely, GPs in the North-West and the East Midlands were less likely to be holding such outside appointments. But even *within* every region except the South-East a higher percentage of doctors in non-designated than in designated areas were engaged in some kind of medical work in addition to general practice. It seems, therefore, not only that such outside appointments were more popular (or more easily obtained) in some parts of the country than in others, but also that doctors in designated areas were in some way precluded or discouraged from accepting them. The explanation does *not* appear to lie in the fact that the pressures of work resulting from large lists were sufficiently great to deny respondents in the designated areas any spare time to engage in other professional activities, for the differences between areas remained even with list size held constant.

A minority of these outside appointments involved hospital posts, but the proportion of respondents holding hospital appointments of one kind or another rose from 37 per cent in the designated areas to 50 per cent among doctors in restricted areas. Not only were outside appointments apparently more easy to come by in the restricted areas (and in non-designated areas as a whole), but a higher proportion of them were likely to involve hospital work.

Direct access to hospital beds

Respondents were asked whether they had direct access to any NHS beds where they retained full responsibility for the treatment of their patients. The form of the question was identical to that used by Cartwright in her national sample survey of GPs in 1964.[3] Cartwright found that 61 per cent of her sample of 415 doctors had access to no hospital beds at all; 27 per cent had access to obstetric beds only; and the remaining 12 per cent were able to care for their patients in other types of beds. The results from the present survey, set out in Table A21, differ somewhat from Cartwright's. The proportion of doctors reporting no access at all to hospital beds was lower, ranging from 51 per cent in the designated areas to only 38 per cent in restricted areas. Moreover, the type of bed available also differed somewhat between practice areas. For the doctor working in a designated area the most common form of care which he was able to provide in hospital was obstetric: more than three-quarters of the designated doctors who reported that they had direct access to hospital beds were limited to obstetric beds only. By contrast, only a little over a third of doctors in restricted areas were confined in their hospital work solely to obstetric cases, the remainder having access, in varying degrees, to surgical, medical and geriatric beds. Conversely, whereas only 10 per cent of all designated doctors had any access to beds other than obstetric, the proportion rose to 39 per cent among the restricted doctors.

These findings are consistent with the earlier conclusion that, even allowing for geographical location and list size, the designated areas appeared to offer fewer opportunities for any kind of medical work outside general practice. Can they be explained by regional factors? Some regions of the country certainly had much better access facilities than others. In the South-West, for example, about 70 per cent of all GPs had some form of hospital responsibility, even if only for the obstetric care of their patients, and at least half of all the doctors in the East and West Midlands and the North-West also reported the opportunity to care for some of their patients whilst in hospital. In Yorkshire/Humberside and the South-East, by contrast, fewer than half the doctors had these facilities open to them, whilst in East Anglia the proportion was as low as 40 per cent (although numbers in this region are small). Such regional variations, however, do not adequately explain the observed differences between the practice areas, for even *within* each region except the North-West and Yorkshire/Humberside the percentage of doctors reporting direct access to hospital beds was higher in the non-designated than in the designated sample.

To complement the factual information about the degree of access to hospital care which the doctors actually enjoyed, they were further asked whether they considered this access to be adequate. Responses were recorded on a four-point scale ranging from 'most adequate' to 'most inadequate', and mean scale scores were calculated by the simple technique of assigning a value of 4 to a 'most adequate' response, 3 to an 'adequate' response, and so on. Two aspects of this analysis merit comment. First, the more access doctors had to hospital beds, the greater was their expressed satisfaction. In the designated sample, for instance, the mean score among doctors who had clinical responsibility for obstetric *and* other beds was 2·8, compared with 2·2 among those with obstetric beds *only*, and 1·8 among GPs with no beds at all. In the non-designated sample the respective scores were 2·8, 2·4 and 1·8. Second, the designated doctors as a whole were less satisfied with their access to NHS hospital beds than the others. The mean scale score for all designated doctors was 2·1 compared with a mean score of 2·4 among those in the non-designated sample. This difference follows logically from the variation between the two samples in the reported degree of actual access.

Direct access to diagnostic facilities

The tendency for doctors in the designated areas to have had rather fewer opportunities than their colleagues elsewhere for working beyond the immediate confines of their practices is further reflected in the greater difficulties which they apparently had in obtaining access to various diagnostic facilities. Respondents were asked whether they had direct access (that is, other than through a consultant or casualty) to each of four diagnostic facilities – full-sized chest X-rays, bone and joint X-rays, bacteriological examination of urine, and glucose tolerance tests. This question was also used by Cartwright who found that 54 per cent of all the GPs in her sample had direct access to all four services.[4] In the present survey the proportions were somewhat higher, ranging from 65 per cent among respondents in designated areas to 76 per cent of those in restricted areas. The mean numbers of services to which doctors reported direct access were 3·3, 3·4, 3·5 and 3·6 respectively in designated, open, intermediate and restricted areas.

Inter-regional variations were much larger. Doctors in the Northern, South-Eastern, South-Western and North-Western regions generally reported a fairly high degree of access to the four listed diagnostic services, whereas those in Yorkshire/Humberside and the West Midlands were less favourably placed. But a comparison between the designated and non-designated samples *within* each region shows, somewhat surprisingly, not only that the slight advantage of the non-designated doctors in this respect had disappeared, but that in most cases it had actually become a disadvantage. For whereas the non-designated doctors were rather better off than the others when the whole country is taken as one unit, they were somewhat worse off within each region except the North and the East and West Midlands, and in some cases appreciably so.

As with the question about access to hospital beds, respondents were then asked to assess the adequacy of their local arrangements with respect to the use of diagnostic facilities on a four-point scale, and, also following the pattern set by the earlier question, there was a clear association between the actual situation in each sample and the doctors' assessments of it. The proportion of doctors rating their degree of access to diagnostic services as 'most adequate' ranged from 39 per cent in designated areas to 52 per cent in restricted areas, and also increased as the number of accessible services accumulated. In the designated sample, for instance, the mean score increased from 2·0 among those who had access to none of the four services to 3·4 among those with access to all four services. In the non-designated sample the corresponding range was from 2·0 to 3·5. Regional variations in the degree of satisfaction were of some significance. Fewer than a third of all the doctors in Yorkshire/Humberside and the West Midlands rated their local arrangements as being 'most adequate' (these also being the two regions in which fewest doctors had direct access to all four services), whilst almost half of those in the Northern, South-Eastern and South-Western regions chose this particular rating (reflecting the fact that these three regions had the highest proportions of doctors with full access).

Communications between hospitals and GPs

With respect to the communication of information from the hospital to the GP when patients are discharged, doctors in the designated areas did not fare any worse than their colleagues in other places. Table A22 is conspicuous for its lack of any overall differences between the practice areas in the respondents' assessments of their local communication systems, although in this case the inter-regional contrasts were greater. The Northern region and East Anglia had high overall scores in both samples (about three-quarters of the doctors in both regions rated their local communication systems as 'very good' or 'good'), whilst scores in the East and West Midlands and the South-West were low. The variations between the two samples *within* each region were generally small, except in the South-West, where the mean score was considerably higher for the non-designated than the designated doctors (2·6 against 2·1).

Post-graduate and in-service training

A traditional criticism of British medical education is that many students, having been trained to a very high degree of clinical competence within the intensive and rarefied atmosphere of the teaching hospital, are thrust out into the community when qualified, and more or less isolated from the centres of teaching and research from which they could and should draw continuing support in the form of post-graduate training, refresher courses and the regular supply of information about new advances in medical science. Several attempts have recently been made to overcome this sense of professional isolation which many family doctors undoubtedly feel, and the growth of post-graduate medical centres throughout the country is perhaps the bravest and most successful innovation of all. But little is known of the doctor's own reactions to these developments, or whether their apparent effectiveness has been evenly felt throughout the different regions and practice areas of the country. Three questions were included in the survey about the opportunities which respondents felt they had for this kind of professional interaction; the results point to the general conclusion that, although the inter-area contrasts were quite slight, the restricted areas were generally felt to have the worst opportunities.

First, respondents were asked to rate their opportunities for taking post-graduate or refresher courses on a four-point scale (Table A23). Proportionately more doctors in the designated and open areas rated their access to post-graduate and refresher courses as 'very good' than did those in the intermediate and restricted areas, and the mean scores show a slight but regular decline as one moves from the designated and open areas through to the restricted areas. There were no differences within the two samples between doctors of different ages in the way they rated their opportunities for further education, and the mean scale scores were virtually identical for doctors with and without higher qualifications, and for those with list sizes above and below 2,600. The inter-regional variations were also small: GPs in the East Midlands, East Anglia and the North-West generally recorded lower mean scores than those in other regions (and they were also less likely to rate their opportunities as 'very good'), but the differences were quite slight.

The second question in this section asked the respondents to rate their contacts with teaching hospitals as 'frequent', 'occasional', 'rare', or 'non-existent'. Table A24 shows the distribution of responses between the types of practice areas, and, as with the previous question, confirms that although the inter-area differences were quite small, doctors in the restricted areas had the least amount of contact with a teaching hospital. Fewer of these doctors reported their contacts as 'frequent' or 'occasional', and correspondingly more rated them as 'rare' or 'non-existent'. The designated areas fell about midway in the range: the responses were more favourable than in the restricted areas, but somewhat less so than in the open or intermediate areas. The same pattern is seen in the mean scale scores for each practice area. The greatest differences in frequency of contact with a teaching hospital were seen between doctors who were and were not practising in the same regions as their own medical schools. In both samples the mean scores for doctors working in the regional vicinity of their medical schools were significantly higher than among those who had left their school regions. A sizeable proportion of the contacts which the respondents mentioned were probably with their own universities, and it is understandable that those remaining near to them should maintain their links more easily than those moving farther afield.

The last question about post-graduate training requested the respondents to rate their contacts with post-graduate medical centres on the same four-point scale. Although for most doctors a contact with a teaching hospital was something additional to that with a medical centre, the reverse was not the case. Thus, whereas most doctors who reported their contacts with teaching hospitals as being 'frequent' or 'occasional' were also in regular touch with a post-graduate medical centre, the majority of those who were in regular association with a centre did *not* report any systematic contact with a teaching hospital. This confirms that the post-graduate centres are in fact largely fulfilling one of their intended functions of providing a centre of medical education for GPs who are geographically isolated from a larger medical teaching centre, and, consequently, a far higher proportion of respondents were in regular touch with one of these centres than with a teaching hospital (Table A25). Some two-fifths of all respondents reported 'frequent' contacts with a centre, and for a further third the contacts were 'occasional'. But, as in the previous question, doctors in the restricted areas were rather worse off than those in other areas: only 38 per cent of them reported their contacts with a post-graduate centre as being 'frequent' compared with, for example, 49 per cent of doctors in designated areas. The distribution of mean scale scores further illustrates the relatively favourable responses of doctors in designated areas. The mean score for these respondents was 3·3, compared with 3·2 among doctors in open areas and 3·1 for those in intermediate and restricted areas.

Comments

In view of the primary aims of the survey to investigate mobility and settlement patterns among GPs, it was impossible to include a full set of questions about contemporary conditions in general practice. The intention has been to collect limited data to use as general indicators or tracers of the various circumstances of GPs in different practice areas. The results discussed in this chapter show that in some respects the doctors in the designated sample were more favourably endowed professionally than those in other areas, in some respects they were worse off, and in yet others they were equally placed. The differences, where they existed, were seldom very large between the different practice areas, and they do not support the assumption that conditions of practice in designated areas are consistently worse than elsewhere.

It seems that although doctors in areas with favourable GP/patient ratios were more closely integrated into the surrounding local medical care systems (especially the hospitals), those in the designated areas were more likely to have professional links with the centres of teaching, research and administration. This is doubtless caused in part by the greater concentration of designated areas around the large urban areas and conurbations where the teaching hospitals are located, but the acceptance of change and innovation may also be swifter in these places than in the more remote and conservative areas away from the hub of the city. The evidence for such a cultural lag is reviewed in the next chapter, which deals with certain practice characteristics.

10 The doctor and his practice

> I like the challenge of eighteenth-century medicine in a region with eleventh-century roads. This is one of the areas left where all-round competence is vital; the nearest hospital is forty miles away; we work with rescue components of all three services. No place for a pen-pusher.
>
> GP in Cornwall

List size

The distribution of principals by list size is given for each region and executive council in the annual reports of the Department of Health and Social Security. The figures from the 1971 report reveal some unexpected discrepancies between the percentage of doctors with lists above 2,500 and the proportion of them in designated areas.[1] In the South-Western region, for example, exactly a quarter of all principals in 1970 had lists above 2,500 and the proportion in the East Midlands was similar (30 per cent), yet the proportions of doctors in designated areas were 8 per cent and 44 per cent respectively in the two regions (see Table A2). How is it possible for two regions to have a similar proportion of practitioners with 'large' lists, and yet to differ so greatly in the relative numbers working in designated areas? The answer is found in the range of list sizes *within* each type of practice area, and since these data are not available in published statistics we must turn to the survey results.

Table A26 shows the range in list size for doctors in each type of practice area. This information was obtained from the sample print-out drawn from the Doctor Index which classifies the average list size for each practice in bands of 100 and 200. Unfortunately the interval limit in the Index does not coincide exactly with 2,500: practices of this size are contained within the band 2,400–2,599, but it was possible to estimate the proportion of doctors in practices with average lists above and below 2,500. The results show a substantial spread *within* each area across the range of list sizes. In the designated areas, for example, about a fifth of the doctors were estimated to be in practices with fewer than 2,500 patients per doctor. In other words, about one doctor in five in designated areas had average practice list sizes below the criterion for designation, and about one in ten was in a practice with an average list below 2,200. Even among doctors actually receiving a designated area allowance in 1968 about a fifth had average practice lists below 2,500, which means that more than £300,000 was paid out in designated area allowances in that year to some 800 doctors in practices below the designated size. This amount will certainly increase under the two-tier allowance.

It is clear from these results that a considerable number of respondents were in practices with lists of a size that fell outside the defining limits of the classification of their areas. The one-fifth of designated doctors with practice lists below 2,500 came into this category, and similar calculations can be made for the other practice areas. Thus in open areas about three-quarters of the respondents fell outside the defining range for this type of area (i.e. between 2,100 and 2,500), and the majority exceeded 2,500, yet still they were ineligible for a designated area allowance. In intermediate areas about four-fifths of the respondents had average practice lists either below 1,800 or above 2,100, and just over half of the restricted doctors had lists above 1,800. These results do not invalidate the arithmetic of the Medical Practices Committee in calculating mean list sizes, nor do they imply an undue delay on the Committee's part in revising the classification of areas as the doctor/patient ratios change; all they show is that by classifying an area on the basis of its *mean* list size, many doctors will have *actual* list sizes outside the defined range for the area. The discrepancy assumes financial significance at the border between open and designated areas, where the allowance is paid to a substantial number of GPs with low list sizes and automatically withheld from an even larger number (i.e. those in open areas) whose individual lists nevertheless meet the criterion for designation.

The phenomenon of doctors with 'small' lists being in receipt of a designated area allowance, though numerically significant, may have fewer policy implications than the converse situation of doctors with 'large' lists (i.e. 2,500 or more) being ineligible for the allowance. It is estimated that in 1968 the allowance was withheld from about 7,500 GPs in practices with average lists over 2,500: in 2,000 cases by virtue of practising in designated areas which had not yet qualified for the allowance, and in 5,500 cases by virtue of practising in a non-designated area and therefore being automatically ineligible.[2] If eligibility for the allowance had been based solely on *personal* list size rather than the average for the area there would thus have been about 6,300 more doctors receiving the allowance in 1968 than was in fact the case – an increase of more than 200 per cent. In fact we argue in Chapter 13 that there are no over-riding reasons why the allowance should be paid on the basis of personal list size, but a large number of GPs must nevertheless be wondering whether the designated areas scheme is a mere fantasy. It is to be expected that where the allowance is given on the basis of an area list size some doctors will be ineligible in spite of exceeding the criterion in their personal lists, but it is surprising to find that as many as seven-and-a-half thousand GPs in England are in such a position.

Partnership size

The survey data revealed some interesting differences between the practice areas in the size of partnerships to which respondents belonged (Table A27). GPs in single-handed practices constituted 17 per cent of respondents in designated areas but 27 per cent of those in restricted areas, and conversely, doctors from larger partnerships (three or more partners) were relatively over-represented in the designated sample. The greater tendency to practise single-handed in restricted areas is no doubt related to the fact that these areas are generally to be found in rural and small-town communities. Single-handed doctors in all areas were relatively over-represented among GPs with very large and very small lists, and under-represented in the middle range between about 1,600 and 3,000 patients. Regional differences in the proportion of respondents in single-handed practice were slight, and failed to account for the lower proportion of single-handed practitioners in the designated areas.

Group practice allowance

The group practice allowance (GPA) was received equally by doctors in each type of practice area. Just over half of all respondents were receiving a GPA at the time of the survey, but the proportion of doctors in single-handed and two-man practices who were receiving the allowance was almost twice as great among the non-designated doctors (40 per cent) as in the designated sample (21 per cent).[3] The allowance was distributed among GPs with varying list sizes in a manner that closely followed the distribution of partnership size: doctors in receipt of the payment tended in both samples to be over-represented among those with medium lists (i.e. between about 1,600 and 3,000) and relatively poorly represented among those with larger and smaller lists.

Health centres

Respondents were asked whether their main or branch consulting rooms were in a local authority clinic or health centre. The replies show that the overwhelming majority of doctors had no connections at all with a health centre, neither their main nor branch surgeries being located there. But the proportion of practitioners who were connected with a centre, either through their main or branch surgeries, was three times as great in the designated as in the restricted areas (12 per cent against 4 per cent), with the open and intermediate areas ranged evenly between (10 per cent and 6 per cent respectively). The greater tendency in designated areas to practise from health centres could be a consequence of any number of a variety of factors ranging from a greater responsiveness to change among doctors in designated areas to the inadequacy and obsolescence of existing premises in these areas (which may be a good reason for building a health centre).

Ancillary help

Respondents were asked to indicate what ancillary help, either full-time or part-time, they had in or attached to the practice. The response categories included: secretary/receptionist; district nurse; health visitor; other SRN/SEN; social worker; and other ancillary help. Table A28 shows that the proportion of doctors reporting no ancillary help at all rose from 3 per cent in the designated areas to 10 per cent in the restricted areas. The difference is quite small, but it remains even when allowance is made for list and partnership size.

The type of ancillary help among those doctors to whom it was available varied little between the practice areas. About one doctor in five in each area had secretarial/receptionist services *only*, two in five had a secretary/receptionist *and* at least one nurse attached to the practice, and about a quarter had these and additional social work help. A slightly higher proportion of doctors in designated than in restricted areas had a nurse working in the practice (65 per cent against 57 per cent), and about a quarter of the GPs in each type of area reported having a secretary or receptionist *and* a nurse *and* some other type of worker attached to the practice. Such a high proportion is cause for suspicion. In a few cases the 'other' worker was identified on the questionnaire as a social worker, but in most instances the doctors merely ticked the 'other' response category available on the questionnaire. We do not therefore know what particular skills these workers brought to the practice: they may possibly have been cleaners.

To complement the factual question about any additional staff which doctors actually had in their practices, they were further asked whether they rated their practices in this respect as 'most adequate', 'adequate', 'inadequate' or 'most inadequate'. The distribution of responses in the two samples was virtually identical, and the mean scale score, calculated by assigning a value of 4 to a 'most adequate' response, 3 to an 'adequate' response, and so on, was 2·9 in both cases. About one doctor in five considered his ancillary help to be 'most adequate', just over half rated it as 'adequate', and only a very small proportion of respondents selected the least favourable category – 'most inadequate'. Although the proportion of doctors choosing the top category ('most adequate') increased in relation to the number and type of staff actually available, it remained fairly low even among those who had secretarial, nursing and other help. Only 27 per cent of these doctors in the designated sample rated their help as 'most adequate', and a fifth considered it 'inadequate'. The corresponding figures in the non-designated sample were 35 per cent and 13 per cent. It is impossible to tell from their replies whether these doctors remained dissatisfied with the *quantity* or the *quality* of the assistance available to them.

Night calls

The final question in this section requested the respondents to indicate the number of nights per week, on average, when they were on call for cases other than obstetrics. The same question had been included in Cartwright's earlier survey in 1964, the results showing that 'a fifth were on call every night, another fifth for five or six nights a week on average, two-fifths for three or four and a fifth for two or less'.[4] On this question, as on several others which were repeated identically from Cartwright's survey, our results differed substantially from hers. Only one in ten of the doctors in the present survey reported that they were generally on call every night of the week, and almost half were required on duty for less than three nights. But, as

Table A29 clearly shows, these proportions varied enormously from one practice area to another, with doctors in restricted areas having by far the least number of free nights available to them. The proportion of respondents generally on call every night was almost four times higher in the restricted than in the designated areas (26 per cent against 7 per cent), and whereas over half (53 per cent) of the designated doctors were on call for two or fewer nights the proportion fell to only 22 per cent in the restricted areas. Respondents in open and intermediate areas were generally in a middle position between these two extremes. The more favourable position of the doctors in designated areas is not explained by regional variations, for the percentage of these doctors on call for less than three nights in the week was higher than in the non-designated sample *within* every region except Yorkshire/Humberside and the West Midlands.

An additional factor associated with night duty is the number of partners a doctor has. Cartwright found that the proportion of doctors on call every night of the week fell from 48 per cent among single-handed doctors to only 8 per cent among those with three other partners, and a similar association was found in this survey. But the factor of partnership size did not explain the variations between practice areas. Whereas, for example, 30 per cent of the single-handed doctors in designated areas were on duty every night, the proportion was 41 per cent among single-handed practitioners in the non-designated sample; and the percentages of single-handed doctors on call for two or fewer nights were 30 per cent and 19 per cent respectively in the two samples. Doctors in larger partnerships were on call for correspondingly fewer nights, and hardly any respondents in practices of three or more partners were on call every night of the week, but *within* each partnership size the differentials remained between the two samples.

Comments

The results of this chapter are important, and will be taken up again in the concluding chapter. Their significance lies primarily in the conclusion that, contrary to much popular belief, and for whatever reasons, the conditions of general practice in designated areas are somewhat more aligned to contemporary notions of good medical care than those in restricted areas. To the extent that multiple partnerships, based on health centres with a full range of ancillary help, and with adequate free time for the GP to study and relax, are accepted as valid signs of good general practice, then the greatest room for improvement is seen in those places with the best doctor/patient ratios. To contrast the designated and the restricted areas is, admittedly, to take the extreme cases, but the other practice areas generally fitted evenly between them, and the variations between the designated and the non-designated samples on most of the questions remained even when a control was introduced for regional location. The variations from one practice area to another are astonishingly consistent, and it is difficult to escape the conclusion that what is observed here represents a faithful reflection of what is actually happening up and down the country.

11 The doctor and his area

My ideal practice would be in a salubrious area with the right middle-class neighbours to consort with, stockbrokers, solicitors, etc.

GP in Essex

There is everything a doctor needs here – fishing, a golf course, walking, not many people.

GP in Devon

We were concerned in Chapter 1 with clearing up some of the confusion which has existed in the past about the objectives of the designated area allowance. The point was made that although the original intention of the allowance was to encourage more GPs to settle in areas which, in terms of doctor/patient ratios, are suffering from a shortage of manpower, the payment has sometimes been regarded as a form of compensation for doctors whose lot it is to live and work in the depressed and unattractive regions of the country. The belief appears to be widespread among the medical profession that the designated areas are, as it were, a kind of third world – worthy to receive general medical services, but scarcely fit places in which sensible people would voluntarily choose to live. The replies of many doctors in the survey confirmed the sharp dichotomy which exists in the minds of many GPs between the underprivileged minority in the designated areas and the rest of the population who lead happier lives. But is the distinction really as sharp as this? Are the designated areas in fact as depressed and unattractive as the stereotypic responses of many doctors suggest?

The question is difficult to answer. How is a socially unattractive area to be defined? One approach might be to draw up a list of area indicators (of housing amenities, educational provision, class and income distribution, open spaces, etc.) and then apply them to designated and non-designated areas, measuring the variations between the two groups. However, quite apart from the practical difficulty that the boundaries of practice areas fail to coincide with any other unit for which statistical data are regularly collected, there is the basic problem that the indicators which we, as investigators, might consider important may be different from those which the doctors themselves would accept. An area may be unfavourably rated on a host of 'objective' indicators, yet be wholly acceptable to the doctors practising there because their desire for, say, an urban working-class environment outweighs the extent to which they perceive such indicators to be negative or undesirable. Even those qualities to which the profession as a whole seems to attach much importance (good housing and educational standards, the availability of cultural and recreational outlets, and the proximity of countryside and coast-line) would presumably be valued in different ways by different doctors. If, therefore, we are considering the attractiveness of an area as a possible motivational factor we must focus on the doctors' *perceptions* of an area rather than on any objective features of it, for it is the subjective impact of a locality that will either attract or repel a prospective practitioner.

At the same time, however, a clear distinction must be made between the subjective appraisals of those actually working in the different areas and the impressions of those who have yet to embark in practice. This chapter is concerned with the ways in which the respondents evaluated their own localities, and it must be acknowledged that people who have lived and worked in a locality for a number of years tend to emphasise the more favourable aspects at the expense, perhaps, of those negative features which might have dismayed them at an earlier date. Ideally this chapter should be concerned with the perceptions of doctors about to enter general practice, for it is largely through these people that the stereotypes about good and bad areas are translated into manpower terms, but the sample did not extend to medical students or qualified doctors at risk of being recruited to general practice for the first time.

The respondents in the survey were presented with five area characteristics, and they were invited to assess their localities for each characteristic on a four-point scale of satisfaction. The characteristics were: educational provision, cultural amenities, shopping facilities, recreational facilities, and housing. The four points on the scale, 'very satisfactory', 'satisfactory', 'poor' and 'very poor', were scored from 4 to 1 respectively, and mean scores were calculated for respondents in each type of practice area. The results, set out in Table A30, show that the mean scores in open and intermediate areas equalled or exceeded those in designated and restricted areas on each characteristic, and that the scores in restricted areas exceeded those in the designated areas only in the case of recreational facilities, which probably reflects the penchant among GPs, revealed in other questions, for rural sports and pastimes. The same trend is reflected in the number of doctors choosing the highest category ('very satisfactory'), although this is not shown in the table. More respondents in open and intermediate areas chose this particular response category for each of the five area characteristics, and the lowest proportion of choices came from doctors in restricted areas for each characteristic except recreational facilities.

Although these results might perhaps have been predicted in the light of our earlier observation concerning the tendency of people to react favourably about their localities, they are nevertheless somewhat surprising. In particular, the low ratings among doctors in restricted areas (which are generally assumed to be the most attractive to doctors) are quite unexpected. Several possible explanations are suggested. One which is consistent with the data presented in earlier chapters is that the restricted areas are in fact less attractive places to doctors in the sense that a majority of GPs, wherever they are working, would rate them less highly than the designated areas on most of the criteria used in the survey. The important factor may be the non-industrialised nature of many restricted areas: they are generally (but not exclusively) located in small towns and rural districts. From this would follow their relative isolation not only from the centres of medical teaching, research and administration, but also from the centres of entertainment, commerce and, probably, education. The availability of suitable housing and recreational facilities, which are less likely to depend upon proximity to a large urban area, were in fact rated just as highly in the restricted as in the designated areas – a point which further reinforces this particular interpretation. An alternative explanation of the facts, however, may be that doctors in restricted areas were, for whatever reason, a more critical breed of men than their colleagues in designated areas, and may consequently have evaluated each question against more stringent standards. They may, in other words, have had a generalised tendency to choose lower ratings, and had they also been invited to evaluate some designated areas, would have rated them even lower than their own practice locations.

It is a weakness of a simple rating technique such as this that there can be no certainty which of these two explanations is the better one, but we are inclined towards the former. There appears to be no over-riding reason why the doctors in the restricted areas should, as a category, adopt more critical evaluative standards, and indeed the earlier evidence shows that they did not uniformly choose lower ratings than doctors in designated areas. In some cases the ratings were higher, and in earlier questions which compared the subjective assessments with more objective measures (for example, with respect to direct access to hospital beds and diagnostic facilities) it was shown that a close association existed between the two sets of replies *within* each sample. None of this is conclusive, but the various pieces of evidence suggest that although the designated areas were generally perceived as less desirable places, socially and environmentally, than the non-designated areas as a whole, they nevertheless compared favourably with the restricted areas alone.

Further analyses of the data indicate that these differences remained even when controlled for age, region, and length of time in practice of doctors in different areas. However, these variables were also themselves in some ways associated with the degree of satisfaction expressed about an area. Older doctors (especially those over 65) often expressed greater satisfaction than younger GPs, although the tendency was more marked in some questions than in others. The evaluation of educational provisions showed a clear gradient in this respect, with the mean scale scores increasing regularly with age, but it is possible that the stage of family development rather than the doctor's age was the important factor in this case. The responses to the question about cultural amenities showed a similar pattern of rising satisfaction with increasing age, but the availability of suitable housing, by contrast, was rated identically by all doctors within each sample, regardless of their age. Broadly similar trends were seen when the scale scores were distributed according to the length of time which the doctors had spent in their current practices. This is to be expected, since age and length of time in practice were themselves positively related. It is, however, interesting to note that, with the exception of educational facilities, there was no consistent tendency for doctors to react either more or less favourably as their familiarity with the area increased.

Doctors in different regions varied quite widely in the degree of satisfaction which they expressed about their localities; but few clear regional patterns emerged from the data. In the designated sample East Anglia ranked lowest of the eight regions on almost all counts (though the frequency in this region is admittedly low), while the North-West, the East Midlands and the South-East each achieved consistently high rankings. In the non-designated sample, on the other hand, the East Anglian doctors were fairly prominent among those expressing favourable responses (along with those in the South-East, Yorkshire/Humberside and the North-West), whilst those in the East Midlands scored low. In sum, it is clear that substantial inter-regional differences did exist in the doctors' ratings of their areas, but that these variations neither explained the better overall ratings in the non-designated areas, nor revealed any complete consistency between designated and non-designated doctors within any region in their evaluation of their localities.

12 The doctors speak

> The GP is in the front line of the battle, but nobody bothers to ask him his opinion about things.
>
> GP in Norfolk

In this penultimate chapter we move from the quantitative approach of previous chapters to a more impressionistic level by considering the doctors' own accounts of some of the factors which have motivated them throughout their careers. The material is drawn partly from the free-answer questions included in the main survey, and partly from tape-recorded follow-up interviews with a selected sub-sample of respondents. The object is simply to illustrate some of the points contained in earlier chapters, and there is no implication that the quotes included in this chapter are in any way representative of all GPs in the survey.

The designated area allowance

There was a fairly widespread feeling of scepticism about the effectiveness of the allowance, although by no means all respondents were hostile to the principle of the payment or wished to abandon the scheme entirely. A substantial number of doctors accepted the need for inducements and agreed in principle with the use of cash incentives, but were critical either of the current amount of the allowance or of the regulations governing its payment. (It must be remembered that at the time of the survey the two-level system had not yet been introduced.) In all, just over a third expressed views about the allowance which were broadly classified as 'favourable', although many also added riders about the scope and administration of the scheme, and several made it clear in their replies that they were judging the payment as a compensation rather than an inducement.

> I am doubtful if the allowance has any great effect in attracting doctors, although it probably provides some compensation to doctors already in the area who are overloaded.

I have sacrificed a larger income to find a more congenial practice and I am pleased that people practising in less pleasant surroundings should get paid more.

Typical of the many GPs who approved the payment in principle but who had reservations about it in practice were these replies:

I think the allowance is reasonable and fair, although with taxation as it is £400 is not enough. The government is already getting doctoring in the designated areas on the cheap, and the strain is so great that an added inducement is needed to encourage more help.

We are all on very full lists (24,000+ between seven of us) and try as we might we can't get another partner on the basis of three months assistantship and three years to parity. If the designated area allowance was more we could offer better financial terms.

Several reasons were suggested why the allowance has been largely ineffective. The most important was simply that £400 made up far too small a proportion of the average GP's income to constitute a realistic inducement.

Financial benefit is little encouragement to the doctor who has an excessive workload, and an additional £400 is hardly likely to attract new doctors into an acknowledged 'difficult' area at a time when entrants to practice have so wide a choice of attractive areas which offer very good facilities medically, and early partnerships on excellent terms.

To be cut off – say, practising in a community of non-whites – this I think is where you need to attract them with money. But £400 just isn't enough for a practice like that where there's no decent medical centre, no night cover and no opportunity to do outside jobs. This to me would be the time when I would need compensating, but a mere £400 wouldn't be enough.

You take Burnley, for example. I was there in 1950. If it's the same as it was then you wouldn't get me there for less than £2,000 a year extra. I'm quite serious – it was a filthy hole.

Most respondents knew about the allowance and some had fairly strong views about it one way or the other (although a few had apparently never heard of it), but the impression was gained that more might be done to publicise the payment among medical students and doctors in their pre-registration year. To the extent that the higher allowance is going to act as any kind of incentive at all it will probably be among younger practitioners and those entering general practice for the first time. The new payments were announced after the main survey had been completed, but there were some indications from the follow-up interviews that younger GPs might take the upper level as a serious inducement. This is a GP of 34:

> At times I suppose just after the income tax has come in you would think yes of course, if you're going to lose £750 worth of income this would be reason enough to make a move. But at other times, when life's okay and you've been enjoying things and nobody's been bloody minded in the surgery, probably not. [Later in the interview] Just to turn over in one's mind the fact of this plus or minus £750 is a most interesting concept.
> Yes. It clicks up a bit on the adding machine.

A second criticism of the allowance, voiced by many practitioners, concerned the disincentives inherent in the scheme. One such disincentive was clearly recognised by the Review Body when, in several reports following the introduction of the allowance, the members refused to recommend an increase on the grounds that, should it be fixed at too high a level, the loss would cause financial embarrassment or even hardship to incoming practitioners when the area ceased to be designated. The responses from the survey vindicate the Review Body's fears, for repeatedly the point was made that no doctor in his right mind would set much store by an incentive that was specifically designed to cease as soon as it succeeded. The continuation of the allowance for a concessionary period of three years was often seen as an irrelevant sop. Closely allied to this was a general dissatisfaction with the three-year qualifying period before the allowance is paid: a doctor moving to a designated area during the qualifying period may well be jeopardising his chances of ever receiving the allowance, and hence the incentive to move is weak.

> This area has been designated for most of my time. When a new doctor enters the place it gets re-classified as open for a few weeks. Thus it has not been continuously designated, and the situation is ridiculous.

> It should be paid during the period of designation, on a yearly basis, and *not* be paid later when the doctor may have moved or

died. The money can then be used to purchase additional time-saving appliances, or to pay locums for extra off-duty, etc.

A more serious disincentive, never considered publicly by the Review Body, is that exerted on the existing practitioners in an area, who have a strong financial motivation to retain their allowance by keeping out newcomers. The temptation probably increases in areas where the average list size is only just above the criterion, where the loss of the allowance would not outweigh the slightly easier work-loads resulting from the introduction of new doctors to the area. Respondents were, understandably, reluctant to talk about this particular disincentive, but there was some evidence that in many designated areas an unwritten agreement exists to retain the classification.

> It produces a situation whereby local practitioners see to it that the area stays designated. It is certainly open to abuse.

> Once an area is designated for three years there is a tendency for established practitioners not to seek a further partner if his employment would cause the designated status of the area to be lost.

Such disincentives are serious and cannot be ignored. They will increase as the value of the allowance rises, and the introduction of the two-level system of payment is likely to add a second point where marginal disincentives are particularly high (i.e. where the average list size is just over 3,000). The Review Body's answer to the problem of disincentives (that the prospect of withdrawal of designation from such areas is remote) not only displays a remarkable lack of faith in its own policies, but is also based on shaky assumptions. Areas *do* become de-designated from time to time, admittedly few to date, but they are likely to do so at an increasing rate in the future for reasons largely unconnected with the allowance (Chapter 2). We discuss various ways by which these disincentives might be removed in the concluding chapter.

A third major criticism of the allowance centred on the arbitrary definitions involved in its administration. Doctors complained about the narrowness of designating an area purely on its average list size, and about the anomalies involved in the arbitrary fixing of medical practice area boundaries.

> I practise on the border of a designated area into which I go to treat many of my patients. Likewise the doctors in the

> designated area without exception have many patients in my area. I consider in my case this is grossly unfair and have even had a personal hearing in London. This principle still rankles a great deal.
>
> I am surrounded by designated areas where strange to say there is little colour problem, few fights at night and few drunks. The morbidity is less than in my area judging from the load of work of my colleagues in these areas whenever I meet them.
>
> The only proper criterion for extra payment is work done related to difficulties encountered. The present assessment is purely theoretical, e.g. by moving our surgery 200 yards down the road we would be paid £1,600 p.a. gross extra for the same workload.

Comments such as these tend to ignore the realities of the situation. It would seem, for example, that GPs who might be eligible for an allowance by virtue of having 60 per cent or more of their patients living in a designated area are not always aware of the possibility, and however the boundaries are drawn there will always be some cases of anomaly and hardship between each side. Nevertheless, there appears to be a strong case for reconsidering the conditions upon which the allowance is contingent, for as well as the difficulties mentioned by the respondents there is the additional problem, quantified in Chapter 10, of GPs with personal lists above 2,500 failing for one reason or another actually to receive the allowance. These points are taken up again in the next chapter, which reviews possible changes in the system of controls and incentives.

Finally, a small section of doctors declared themselves opposed to the allowance in principle.

> My area is designated. I feel that the number of patients in my practice [partnership of two] is huge, and we have to work very hard, day and night. We do our best to provide the best possible medical service. It is very strenuous physically and mentally. I do not think an extra payment of £400 is the answer to this problem. I personally do not think that even £1,000 is the real answer. The principle is wrong. I would very much like to reduce the number of patients and provide a better medical service.

In most cases the objection appeared to represent a specific example of a more fundamental hostility to the whole concept of a National

Health Service. One doctor, for instance, described the allowance as 'a pathetic attempt to treat a symptom, not the cause', another said it was 'a terrible indictment of the Health Service that such an allowance is needed at all', and a third described his feelings about the payments as 'quite unprintable'. The politically oriented responses are typified in this answer:

> I consider this unfair, as I believe in a free-floating market, with restoration of the right to buy and sell practices as before 1948. Such a problem would not then arise.

The choice of a practice area

If financial incentives have not in the past been much of an inducement, on what grounds did the doctors in the survey select their practice locations? The earlier analyses indicated three potent factors: the market situation, especially in the 1950s and early 1960s, when GPs took almost any post offered in order to secure a living; the existence of prior connections with the area through family ties; and the existence of professional contacts. Do the doctors' own explanations cast any further light upon the matter?

Social and family ties

In response to the question 'What influenced your choice of this area as the one in which to practise?' the two most commonly cited factors were social or familial links, and professional contacts. Each was mentioned by at least a fifth of the respondents. Family and social connections were listed more frequently by designated than by restricted doctors, and, partly reflecting this, were also more significant factors in the choice of area among doctors in the north than in the south. Sometimes the family influences were also bound up with professional considerations.

> Strong family ties – my father and grandfather before him had been in general medical practice in this area, which I consequently knew well before entering practice here myself.

> My father-in-law was in practice here: he had been working far harder than I ever had during the war, he had had a terrible war and was tired out, and he said 'I want you to come right away, I can't go on much longer.' So I came.

But most respondents who mentioned the importance of family ties did not have these reinforcing motives of family background.

> When I entered general practice despite many applications I only heard from two, one in Bristol and one in Sheffield. I chose this one because having qualified here I had many friends, and it was near my home and my wife's home.

> I'm a Durham man and consider I understand the Durham miner and his ways, and these form the bulk of my practice.

Of particular interest in this context is the influence which a wife has on her husband's decisions about when to move and where to settle. Chapter 8 explored the relationship between a doctor's current practice area and his wife's home area, and it was shown that the influence is roughly on a par with that of the medical school. It was clear from the interviews, however, that although many doctors had not in fact chosen to settle in their wives' home areas, most had regarded them as equal partners in decisions about moving.

> I think that if anybody is making a move, the place should be assessed by the wife in the first instance. I would say that this is the most important advice I could pass on to young doctors, let the wife assess the new place first.

In some instances, in fact, the wife's views seem to have been the dominant ones.

> I think I had as much influence as a wife should have on her husband. At that time it was a mental hospital or divorce, so I suppose it was fairly strong. *I* scanned the *BMJ*, *I* sent for the forms, *I* filled them in, and *he* signed them. We were both in agreement that we should move, and I went through the *BMJ* with a toothcomb and did everything.

More commonly, a wife's difficulties were the basis for a joint decision to move.

> My wife didn't get on with my senior partner. He used to swear at her over the phone. He expected her to be there all the time to answer the phone. She was out in the garden one day hanging up nappies and was a long time answering the phone and he was quite abusive to her. Well, she was unhappy, so we decided to leave. I applied for some posts in Scotland to please my wife.

The way in which the decision processes within a family change over time is well illustrated by this GP's wife in the East Midlands:

> When we came here it was primarily John who decided; he was the one who was going to be working in whichever area it was. I came down of course and I saw the house and I saw the area and was happy to come, but I don't think the decision was really mine. But if we are going to move now it would be a family decision. There's all sorts of things, schools, and all amenities to be taken into consideration as well. Ten years ago it was different.

Professional contacts

Together with family ties, professional contacts were the most commonly mentioned reason for the choice of practice location. Unlike family connections, however, which were more significant for doctors entering designated than non-designated areas, the importance of professional contacts was stressed equally by doctors in each type of practice area. Some cases that were classified under this heading were highly individualistic:

> A tip from my brother, a GP in New Zealand, that the senior partner here was 83 and contemplating retirement. I carried the old B. on my back for four painful years.

Much more typical were these cases, which also illustrate the significance of the siting of medical schools.

> I had been attached to this practice for several weeks in my final year at medical school, as an introduction to general practice.

> I had completed a period as surgical registrar at the local infirmary just before joining the practice. The other two principals were well known to me, and recognised in S. as very good clinicians.

Practice facilities

The third most frequently mentioned reason for choosing a practice location, cited equally by doctors in each type of practice area, was some aspect of the practice itself.

> I chose the *practice* – the area was decided by chance. It was a group practice with good hospital facilities and the possibility of anaesthetic sessions.

> An attractive advertisement specifying: 1. Rural area, 2. Dispensing practice, 3. Expanding practice, 4. Interest in scientific medicine. Discovered at interview: 1. The obviously high standard of medicine practised by the principal, 2. The fact that he would make an excellent senior partner (he did, and did better still by resigning after four years), 3. The availability of hospital sessions, 4. Access to diagnostic facilities.

Younger doctors were generally more influenced by these considerations than older ones, and it is likely that entrants to general practice will increasingly be attracted by efficient and well-run partnerships, with adequate supporting services and opportunities for hospital work etc. Some of the older doctors in the survey deprecated this trend, arguing that modern aids and facilities do not add to a man's competence as a family doctor and can only serve to attract second-rate practitioners seeking to hide their inadequacies behind an aura of scientific medicine; but this was a minority view. Much more common was the opinion that money spent on improving practice conditions in the unattractive areas would have a much greater effect in attracting doctors to such places than a fairly small financial carrot, but such opinions seemed often to rest on the assumption that practice conditions are invariably and uniformly worse in the designated areas.

Chance and constraint

The next most frequently mentioned factor in the choice of a practice location involved chance, constraint or some form of involition. The replies gave the strong impression that GPs in designated areas were much less likely than their colleagues elsewhere to have chosen their practices for positive, volitional reasons; rather, their answers consistently reiterated the theme that they had little choice in the matter, or that this was the only vacancy offered at a time when a job was quickly needed. Typical of such replies are the following.

> Joined practice in 1950. 90 applicants. Short-listed in London. Dam' lucky to be accepted.

> No choice at all. No money – could not have paid removal

> expenses – and two babies. In a full-time industrial medical officer's post as an assistant with no hope of promotion and bored to death. At that time [1953] there was an artificial surplus of doctors and jobs were hard to come by. I was offered a partnership on a very thin financial basis and took the chance. I continue to this day to live by courtesy of the Bank Manager.

> At that particular time (I'm talking about 1953) it was nothing to apply for fifty vacancies and not even get shortlisted. In this case I rang the man up and he told me that 200 people had applied. That meant they weren't going to get it and would have to apply elsewhere. Eventually I got an assistantship (in a seaside town) and after twelve months they offered me a view.

> When I was looking for a job it didn't worry me where I went. The reason I happen to be here is that I applied to this Executive Council, and to about twenty-nine others. I was interviewed for about twelve jobs; five times in Liverpool and twice in Sussex. The only reason I'm here is that I happened to get the job here. The next job might have been in Lancashire, and I'd have been there.

The enormous surplus of doctors relative to vacancies in the 1950s undoubtedly created a climate of competition and uncertainty that is unlikely to recur within the next decade at least. For a large number of doctors their choice of where to practise was simply not a choice in a volitional sense: it was a solution forced upon them and, often, gratefully accepted despite harsh or detrimental terms.

Environmental factors

The last set of factors mentioned by a significant number of doctors as a reason for choosing their practice locations concerned the general environment. In a few cases there was a strong preference for an urban environment, but for most doctors the ideal was open countryside, with fishing and shooting facilities, and a small practice of loyal and uncomplaining country folk with a proper respect for the position of the family doctor. The proportion of respondents who reported choosing their current practices mainly for their rural properties increased from about one in ten in the designated areas to nearly half in restricted areas, almost all of whom were in the west country or East Anglia.

> Having been born in Somerset and living a greater part of my formative years in and around Exmoor and being very interested in all country pursuits, it was only natural that I should seize the opportunity to return when this idyllic rural practice became available.

> It is a quiet, rural area with a small market town and modest inland resort as its centre. The population is fairly stable, of varied type but with no extremes of poverty or affluence. We are within reasonable distance of family connections, the Welsh mountains and the Welsh coast. We are surrounded by unspoilt country of great beauty.

> Having done locums in town and country practices I felt I could not tolerate normal impersonal town practice. After searching for months for a country practice with a nice period house I eventually found this place and was offered the vacancy by the Executive Council.

The theme of escaping from the suffocation of the cities ran strongly through the declared motives of rural doctors – especially those in the west country, many of whom had formerly practised in urban settings. The yearning for the peace and quiet of rural practice probably explains the concentration of restricted areas in regions and counties with low urban densities, notwithstanding the financial loss that is involved in taking a smaller list and the greater isolation from large medical centres. There were signs, however, that younger doctors placed greater emphasis on professional satisfaction than on environmental solitude, and it is likely that in future they will be more attracted by recent innovations in the structure of general practice (for example the tendency towards group practice, health centres, the employment of ancillary staff, increasing contacts with hospitals, the use of more sophisticated equipment etc.) than by the joys of small rural partnerships, lacking as they do many of these modern aids and innovations.

Some case histories

To illustrate some of the diverse routes through which GPs have entered their current practices three case studies are presented. They are not claimed to be typical in any sense – indeed they have been deliberately selected for their particularly interesting (and therefore unusual) features – but they usefully illustrate the complex interaction of events which determine the geographical orientation of family doctors. The studies are based on edited extracts from the tape-recorded interviews, and certain details have been eliminated or falsified to preserve the doctor's anonymity. Each doctor has given permission for his story to be published.

Dr A., practising in the west country

> One day after the results came out in medical school a friend said where are you going to live? I said I don't care, as long as it isn't a teaching hospital. I had general practice in mind from the word go, so I knew the widest experience was to be had in general hospitals. He said I am off to Lancashire, how about joining me? So I just went off to Lancashire. I remained there for two years. It was an excellent experience because I literally worked in all hospital departments. As house surgeon you did gynaecology and eyes as well. As house physician you have the VD beds and the skin beds. As casualty, well you are the all-rounder in the hospital. It was very, very good experience. The hospital had 200 beds and it carried just the right basic work for general practice. From there I went to a maternity hospital in the midlands because I wanted a D.Obst., and I was given a great deal of work that would normally have been done by registrars or senior registrars. I did eight months obstetrics and then went on to do paediatrics in the north-east. And then a short time after I had finished my paediatrics I went to the orthopaedic hospital as anaesthetist looking for a post in general practice. The big fact when I applied for a new practice was nothing to do with medicine – I didn't drive. So one or two practices that I looked at said well sorry, old boy, if you can't drive you're not much good to us. That was why I had to turn down an assistantship in Cumberland. I was interviewed for other practices: there was one at Newcastle and one near Durham. That was an awful place, rows and rows of council houses and this doctor's house almost in the middle of them. We arrived on a Sunday afternoon, and he was obviously interviewing several people. We sat in the dining room along with all the others. The previous assistant told us that he had been thrown out, and that the principal was having a series of assistants. It was a very curious set-up, the man was an alcoholic or something, and we didn't go there.

Then I was asked to go back to Lancashire where I'd done my first hospital job. It was a contact I had made through the hospital, but I wasn't very keen. It's a sleepy place, a very large Jewish community and people who come from the cotton towns. There was quite a lot of private practice but the place was over-doctored, and the opposition was strong. Eventually I got an assistantship with view in the midlands. I took it because it was the only place where the partner presented the earnings for the practice and said your future here is extremely secure. He said I would inherit the private patients and the factories which were extremely lucrative. He was offering £200 more than the average at the time, a large Victorian house with eight bedrooms and a car. I had no money at all at this time, so beggars can't be choosers. It was obvious from the moment I got there that I would have to run the practice despite the fact that he was the senior man. He did four half days a week and disappeared to the West Indies every winter, so I was literally running a one-man show, covering everything. Looking back we were absolute fools, we fell for the lot.

And my wife was unhappy from the moment we arrived. [*Mrs A:* It was so dismal and drab, and I became depressed. One day was exactly like the last and I knew tomorrow would be exactly the same again and I couldn't look forward to anything. All I could see was the year ahead being exactly the same as the past one.] After three or four years it became very obvious to me that my wife would not settle there, and from about the fourth year we started looking for other practices. It became almost an obsession, so much so that I applied for practices that I knew I would damn well hate. It was quite a situation to be in, living in an environment to which neither of us was accustomed. I was from Scotland and my wife from the south-west and there we were in the industrial midlands. When we started looking for practices my wife was mad keen on Edinburgh, and I must have looked at five or six practices in Edinburgh over the years. But I wasn't all that keen. You know what Edinburgh is like, tall terraced houses, I didn't fancy that. I was offered three practices in Edinburgh and turned them all down, mainly because the houses were not what I wanted. The practices were in many ways suitable but the housing situation wasn't. We had also got used to running a large practice with a good income so we had got used to a standard of living that no practices that we looked at in Scotland could provide. We liked to wine and dine a bit. We also looked at two practices in Aberdeenshire, but they didn't appeal to me because one of them involved running a maternity clinic of approximately 100 beds single-handed, which meant a lot of night work which I didn't fancy. The other thing that put me off was when I stopped at a place and asked a man if he could direct me to the late doctor's house (this was a death vacancy). He gave me full directions but I didn't understand two words he said. I said to my wife we won't bother to see the widow, I can't understand a word they say. I had really set my sights on a seaside or country practice as my ideal, and of course this was the pattern before the war when you were prepared to spend ten years in an industrial practice to acquire the capital to buy a practice in a nice seaside town. I saw no reason whatsoever why the Health Service should change this practice. We applied for practice after practice in the south-west and never got short-listed. I could never understand this. If you weren't short-listed the executive council told you who had been appointed, and we used to look pop-eyed at these letters which came; and I would go off to the public library and read the qualifications of these people, and they weren't nearly as good as mine. We decided that perhaps my accent was wrong.

Well, we looked at these practices regularly for about six years, in Devon and Cornwall to start with but then in Shrewsbury, Sutton Coldfield, another two in Warwickshire, and several in the Birmingham area. Then things finally came to a head just before my partner retired. We had this enormous house, you see, and I had bought a half share in it. The senior partner had had two other partners before I joined the practice, and the house was divided into two, with one partner living in each end of the house. Then out of the blue one day, without telling us, this family of father, mother and child arrived, asking for the key to get into the flat, whilst he was on holiday. [*Mrs A:* I was about seven months pregnant and I sobbed my heart out. It was a terrible experience, you know, it was getting dark about seven, it was in October, and the man knocked at the door and said 'Can I have the key?' and I said 'What key?' He said 'To the flat next door,' so I said 'What are you going to do?' I had visions of alterations or something, and he said 'We are moving in,' and I asked 'Who's we?' He said 'My wife and child and myself.' That was the end as far as I was concerned, and I remember they moved in on the Saturday, I saw this van arrive and it knocked down the cable for the lights to the garage. Mother came along too and knocked at the door and said which is my daughter's clothes-line. I said neither, they both belong to me. It was a nightmare.] Then he converted the outhouses into four garages, and we had people whizzing in and out of the back in their cars with little toddlers running around. And then the coloured people started to come in, and all in all that was the beginning of the end.

I started applying far more intensely for practices at this time, but by this time I was getting a bit more choosy, and I said to myself, if I am making a move I might as well make a real move. And it was at this time that a friend in South Africa kept pestering me, why not come and join me, I'm making £20,000 and I will give you a half share. He phoned at eight o'clock one day all the way from South Africa and said for God's sake come and join me here, so I said to my wife shall we go and have a look at it? I had serious reservations as to whether she would like it, but she said all right, let's get out of here anyway and go and have a look at it. There was a lot of trouble selling the house because the new man hadn't got any capital and couldn't raise a mortgage, and the council would only give him a £5,000 mortgage. So I attended a council meeting and I said well, to help you out (because otherwise the place would have been without a doctor) I am prepared to sell the house for £5,000, which means my making a loss of about £2,500. They said, well this is fantastically good of you, and they gave him the mortgage for it then. But we didn't do too well out of it.

We arrived in South Africa with the temperature well over 100, and I could see my wife wasn't really taken by this. And within a very short while it was obvious that my friend didn't really want me in with him because he was always showing me advertisements of practices in Durban and he kept saying, I would recommend you to go and look at these. We then discovered that he had already asked three other people out on the same pretext, but after nine years he still hadn't taken a partner. We could never work this one out at all because, as I said, he had even telephoned me at eight o'clock one morning to ask me to join him. He was making about £24,000 a year and he hoped that in subsequent years it would exceed £30,000, and we think his reason for asking us to go was probably something as trivial as showing us how well he had done. Well, we came back very quickly, taking a holiday cruise on the way, and we stayed with my wife's relatives in the south-west. By this time I was quite certain I did not want to practise again in an industrial area, that it would have to be a country practice, so I was quite prepared to do locums for a long spell.

I started off as a locum in a holiday camp in the north of England, which was an absolutely killing job, believe it or not, because of the numbers involved. Then someone who knew us in the midlands wrote to say he was forming a group practice and would we go and join him. He offered £100 a week while I was making up my mind. I said I don't suppose for one moment I shall join you because I spent twelve years there and was only too glad to get out; but I'm quite happy to have £100 a week while I'm deciding. So we went there, and then several executive councils in the area heard that I was back again in the midlands and instead of me applying for practice vacancies I was getting the clerks of the councils ringing me up saying will you come and practise in our town. But we really felt at this stage, having taken the enormous step of going to South Africa, that if we didn't make our stand then we never would. Well, after that job I had another locum in Staffordshire, and I also looked at two posts in Scotland, but we just didn't have the money at that time to buy the houses or premises. Then there were these two jobs going in the west country so I applied almost as a matter of routine. After applying we went down to visit my wife's mother for a weekend and we came and had a look at this one, but we weren't at all inspired. My wife has always been attracted to the bright lights, and she was wondering what on earth she would do with herself. A little while later we were saying that we should have heard by now who got those two practices, and blow me the post came, and it was a letter from the Medical Practices Committee asking me to be interviewed in London on the Wednesday. I'd never heard of such a thing in my life: I thought there was something fishy about the practice. I asked some colleagues for their advice and they said I might as well go. So with a very casual letter, because this was a very foggy time, I said if the fog isn't too bad I shall appear before your Committee; if it is very foggy I shall not appear.

It was a lovely sunny day on the Wednesday, so off I went. Two were there to be interviewed, we had both recently returned from abroad, and the other one had connections in this part of the world; so he was well placed. He was in with the Committee for half an hour, and he came out sweating. He said, they've got tabs on you, they know every move you've ever made in your life in there. I asked whether they knew about his being in Canada (because he hadn't told them) and he said yes. But they rattled through my interview in five minutes, and then they called me back and said, well, Dr A. it's the unanimous decision of this Committee that you are the best man to fill this vacancy. Will you accept? I said yes. One of them then said don't do anything yet because there will almost certainly be an appeal. Well, an appeal was duly lodged by the executive council over the Committee's decision to appoint a doctor over the heads of the local people and in preference to a local candidate; but the Minister turned it down, so here we are.

Dr B., practising in the East Midlands

After I qualified I was allowed one year in house jobs until I had to do my national service, so I went into the Air Force for a couple of years, but wanting ultimately to do general practice. Prior to demob I started getting phone calls from a practice in Sussex asking if I would go down as a trainee assistant for a year. It had been my home, so there was no problem of accommodation, and that's where I did my assistantship. In fact I stayed in Sussex for fifteen months because I started at the beginning of a summer spell, and at the end of the twelve months the partner asked me if I would stay on and cover the holidays. I'd been applying for jobs for the last nine months, but didn't have anything, so I stayed.

When I got down to the last three months the Practice Bureau started sending me things. I was applying all over the shop in the south, but I wasn't even shortlisted. They didn't want to know me. The second holiday spell finished and we set off up to our home in Lancashire on a fortnight's holiday with pay, to find, on arrival, that a letter had been dropped in earlier by a doctor in the town. His partner, who had been my wife's family doctor for years and years had died about a year previously, and poor little Dr M. had been struggling along on his own. He had had one or two assistants who just didn't work out; either they were unsatisfactory from the working point of view, or, lending them one of his cars, they wrote it off. He hadn't had a holiday since his partner had died. I found this note, if I hadn't got anything fixed up and I was at a loose end would I be interested? So I went round and within a week I had started. But I was still applying for jobs. We had one child and wanted to increase the family, but I thought it wouldn't be fair until we had settled somewhere. So I went on applying, with a testimonial from Dr M. to add to the Sussex testimonial. You see, there was no chance of a partnership in that practice. The old partner, who had been my wife's family doctor, had got a son struggling through finals at Manchester and kept failing, and the old boy on his deathbed made Dr M. promise to keep the practice open for his son. So after I had been with him for a bit Dr M. said, I'd like you to stay for ever, you go down very well here, but I must keep my promise. He didn't stand in my way when I was applying.

We looked at lots of places. One week we were in Hampshire and a fortnight later in Nottinghamshire. But even when I had been shortlisted I either heard nothing or got a stereotyped note saying thank you for coming over etc. but the post has been filled by a friend of one of the partners. I wanted to go south, somewhere near the sea, but thought I was reaching out of my depth to get there. Earlier the Practices Bureau had warned me that the average waiting time from getting on their books till getting settled was two years, and people wanting to go south were waiting up to five years. We nearly got several posts but they were filled by friends or relatives. It went on and on like that and then a vacancy came up in the south-east with an Indian doctor. Well frankly I couldn't care less who a person is if you get along all right and like them. So I went down for an interview and he seemed a nice chap. He presented the practice in glowing terms, growing in numbers, etc., so down I went. He took me on instantly. But within a fortnight of starting only three people had turned up at the surgery. A request for a house call came in only about twice a week, and altogether this didn't add up to a practice of three and a half thousand and growing. The trouble was I couldn't get him pinned down. He had a brother running a restaurant up in London, and most evenings he would go up there and then the next day he'd be sleeping it off. After a fortnight I went in to the Clerk of the Executive Council and said, 'Look, what is the position?' He said, 'Well,

I am not allowed to divulge this.' I said, 'I know you aren't officially, but I have in fact come down here with the intention of being an assistant with view to partnership and I can't pin Dr H. down into bringing me in. But it all sounds very, very wrong to me that the practice is being grossly misrepresented, and I would just like your confirmation one way or the other.' And he said, 'All right, under those circumstances I will tell you. The numbers for months have been dropping at the rate of 80 a week, the practice is now under 2,000 and still dropping.' I then confronted Dr H. the next time we linked up, and he agreed that this was in fact the case, but he wanted me to stay and offered me instant partnership. I said the numbers left aren't really enough to support one let alone two and he said 'Well, if you stay you can have the whole of the take.' I said that was stupid. He didn't even own his own house, and he was renting surgery accommodation underneath his furnished flat. So I said, 'I'm awfully sorry, I like it here, but there's no future for two doctors in this practice.' Then I rang back to Dr M. in Lancashire and asked if he'd got another assistant yet. He said no. I asked why not and he said 'I've been waiting to get a phone call from you.' So back I went. My wife had been there all the time (I'd been staying in a guest house in the south-east) and so we had smiles and handshakes all round. The old partner's son had failed his finals again, I started applying all over again, and it was like old times.

I applied for about five town practices altogether in a bunch. I basically wanted a town practice in a partnership, but not in a city – not London or Birmingham. I'd seen enough of these lone wolves scratching around, no time off, wives acting as receptionists. I wanted to get into a partnership and climb up with time. This practice was one of the five and one evening there was a phone call from the senior partner asking us to come over on the Sunday. I said I would be delighted, but I would first have to check with Dr M. because he might have made alternative arrangements. But the senior partner wasn't listening: he just breezed on. 'We'll see you at 11 o'clock at such-and-such a place. Cheerio!' Immediately the phone went again; it was Dr M. 'Have you just had a call from Dr S. in — ?' Yes. 'Well, the crafty old devil must have booked a couple of rapid calls and asked for me to be blocked while he was ringing you. He's just told me you're going over on Sunday!'

So we came over and were taken for a quick drive round. We were given a meal at the Midland Hotel, looked at the surgery house, this, that and the other, and then went back to have tea with the other partners. Before we left the senior partner turned up again and said 'We'd like to have you but you must start a week today. If you can't come we'll get somebody else.' Just like that. So I came over the following Sunday and moved into the surgery house with the previous assistant and his wife for ten days until they moved out. We'd scarcely heard of the place before we came here. We accepted more or less on the spur of the moment that Sunday. All we wanted was to get settled, and we didn't mind where it was then. We only wanted the house and the job. We had never thought of the people or what things were really like.

Dr C., practising in the West Midlands

While I was finishing my pre-registration jobs I was looking in the journals for a suitable trainee post. I wanted to be a GP and I wanted to go into practice with a traineeship behind me. There was nothing in the area of my hospital so I had a free choice of the country. I was married a year before I was qualified and although we both come from Manchester, we were not committed to that area in any way. We thought we would like to try further south. We had some friends in the midlands, and when we visited them for weekends we often thought how splendid it would be to live within easy reach of them. We had the idea then that the 'county town' type practice would best suit our 'image', somewhere in the band of country between Shrewsbury and Leicester, and Gloucester and Luton.

In the *BMJ* there was a traineeship advertised in Oxfordshire, which I applied for. The doctor there was delighted that someone from the north had applied and he made me very welcome. I spent a most pleasant year with him and then started looking for a good assistantship.

We began looking in the area from Hereford across to Leicester, south of Birmingham and preferably on the Worcestershire side. Every week I went through all the advertisements in the *BMJ* that were possibilities. There were perhaps twenty to thirty jobs each week. I had a duplicated 'curriculum vitae' and I sent a copy with a covering letter to each advertisement that interested us. I also approached the Medical Practices Bureau in London, and through them I heard of an assistantship in Nottinghamshire. I went for an interview there. It was a mining village and the doctor's house was an old mansion, standing in beautiful grounds with a small bungalow at the entrance. I was offered the job, and told that I would be living in the bungalow, but we couldn't see it at that time as it was occupied. I was not getting any response to my applications and I had not enough capital to remain unemployed so I was in no position to turn it down. We spent all our spare time – and money – making the place habitable, for the first few weeks after we moved in. The bungalow we were put into was disgusting, and we had to spend about £300 on it. It hadn't been touched for twenty years. It was filthy – not just not decorated but filthy – and we disinfested it of its silverfish, cockroaches and its sundry mice and put in new fireplaces, stripped the bathroom out, well, we had got to live there. We recouped some of our money in salary I suppose, but he got a very nice bungalow out of it. The area wasn't what we had expected, either. It was a drab mining practice in a drab mining area, and as far removed from a 'county town' atmosphere as it was possible to get. After about four months, and several disagreements with the principal over gross inequalities in the duties in the practice, I started to look for another post.

I was getting a bit more experienced. I had an interview in Worcestershire and another in Staffordshire. The doctors there had the area buttoned up, it was a monopoly organisation, and they also ran a little hospital. It was very nice, but it was a condition of entry into the practice that we bought the retiring partner's house at £8,000. All we could raise in loans was about £1,500. We didn't hear any more about that practice. I also went for an interview in Manchester, but I was eventually offered and took an assistantship with view in Herefordshire. We were only there a few months, because it became increasingly clear that I would never be offered the partnership. I was the eighth or ninth tenant of the post, and partnership had never been offered to any of them.

We had to do something other than abortive assistantships, so I thought that by doing locums instead of assistantships I would get better known among GPs in an area. I was struck by the casualness of it all. You finished one locum and then you met another doctor, and it all seemed to be very friendly and casual. I certainly found that doing locums I got a much better insight into what a practice was like, through the patients and through their general attitude towards the practice. They'd got the practice weighed up far better than ever I could in a short period of time, and I soon rumbled that this was a very good way of judging a practice. I did quite a lot of locums – in North Wales, Manchester, Cheshire, Derbyshire, London, Herefordshire, Cheshire again and Staffordshire. It was a hand-to-mouth existence; you would do one job for a fortnight or a month, and at the end of the month you were often still looking for a job to follow on. And all the time I was still applying for interesting practice vacancies, and single-handed practices advertised by executive councils.

I was short-listed for several posts, and when I talked to the other candidates I found that they were having the same difficulties in obtaining a career post. My two university friends also found this period very frustrating, and they both went to Australia, where the different situation enabled them to choose positions that suited them. I was interviewed for two jobs in Lancashire, both on the same day. The morning interview was for a vacancy where the doctor had been struck off. I was offered that one on the spot but I turned it down because I was confident of getting the second job – a death vacancy which I was already temporarily filling as a locum. In fact I was talking to one of the other applicants, a prison doctor, and he felt he was really wasting his time because the sitting tenant always got these vacancies. But in the end he got it, not me. This was all on the same day. I had to make the first decision in the morning (the one I turned down); they wouldn't let me wait until the afternoon to see if I got the death vacancy.

There were other interviews, but this practice I am now in was the only one I was offered. There were seventy applicants for it when it was advertised twelve years ago. It was about my thirtieth application for an Executive Council post and the fifth for which I had been short-listed. It took me from January 1955 until June 1958. You simply cannot talk about *choosing* an area under these conditions.

13 Under-doctored areas: an assessment of current policy

If we do nothing about it, others outside the profession will, and it would be surprising indeed if we found their solutions to our liking.

Dr E. Townsend (*Medical World*, September 1969)

The designated areas: concepts and objectives

We begin this concluding chapter with an appraisal of the basic philosophy of the designated areas. It seems clear, in the first place, that a number of crucially important concepts have not always been explicitly defined and have therefore been used in conflicting and ambiguous ways. The failure to distinguish between the supply of general practitioners and inequalities in their spatial distribution is a major example. One source of this confusion is seen in the BMA's tendency to interpret a rise in the number of designated areas as evidence of an increasingly uneven distribution of doctors.[1] Another source stems from the Office of Health Economics publication, *The Personal Health Services* (1963), which included a chart showing the number of patients residing in each type of practice area from 1952 onwards.[2] Open and intermediate areas are described in the chart as ones of 'balanced distribution', and the commentary states that 'since the mid-1950s there has been less progress in obtaining a better balance in the distribution of doctors'. The same chart was repeated in the Royal College of General Practitioners' survey of the present state and future needs of general practice in 1970, and the same conclusions were drawn.[3] The chart has been used most recently by Clarke, who comments that 'attempts to distribute general practitioners more evenly have met with little success since 1963 [because] the number of people living in designated areas has risen from 9 million in 1963 to 18 million in 1968'.[4]

It is, however, a matter of common sense that 'even-ness of distribution' relates to the *variability* of list sizes over the country, not to the actual number of patients per doctor. An increasing proportion of patients in designated areas *might* indicate a growing imbalance in distribution, but might equally be a sign of a decreasing stock of family doctors relative to the population. If every practice area in the country had an average list of 3,000 the total supply of GPs would be distributed with perfect equality, even though the entire population would be in heavily designated areas. It is clearly possible to have a situation in which the range between areas with very large and very small list sizes is narrowing, yet where overall list sizes are large and rising. To some extent this happened in England during the 1960s. If the average list for the entire country is only a little below 2,500 then quite small deviations from an even distribution could result in moderately large numbers of designated areas. That may well be a sign that more doctors are needed in the system, but it cannot be taken as *prima facie* evidence of an increasing imbalance.

Even when it is clear that certain areas really do suffer a relative deprivation of medical manpower, the method by which the movement towards a desired solution is assessed must be clearly specified. The ultimate objective of existing policies would be a situation in which each practice area had a more or less equal number of patients per doctor and where that number was below 2,500. If this ideal were ever achieved then the need for the designated area allowance in its present form would disappear. Progress towards such a situation, however, may emphasise one of these two components at the expense of the other, and it is therefore a matter of some importance that the relative value of each is clearly stated. Is evidence of an increasing equalisation of list sizes across the country valued more or less highly than a decline in the proportions of doctors or patients in designated areas? Until there is agreement on this basic question much of the current confusion about existing policies is likely to remain.

It would be easier to understand what was happening if trends in the *movement* (as well as the *distribution*) of medical manpower could be monitored. The point was made in Chapter 2 that changes in the number of doctors in any area may result from the interaction of several different processes, yet existing statistics merely show these net changes and give no indication of the varying situations underlying them. A useful first step towards a clearer understanding of the total picture would be a new analysis of relevant data which are already collected by the Department of Health and Social Security, and which could be presented regularly in an appropriate fashion. An ongoing monitoring system of this kind would not only permit an evaluation of policies aimed at affecting the dispersion of family doctors, but might also be of value in the early identification of potentially undesirable trends, suggesting areas in which action might be taken to forestall a future pattern of chronic manpower shortages.

The basic mechanism for such a system already exists, for much of the information contained in Chapters 5 and 6, for instance, is already collected on a routine basis and stored in the Doctor Index. This Index, which is compiled and held by the Statistics Division of the Department of Health and Social Security, contains certain details, including residential location, of all principals and assistants engaged in National Health Service practice. The information is stored in written documents and on punch cards, and new documents and cards are raised for doctors who are admitted to the Medical List for the first time and for those who change executive councils. The *mechanism* of up-dating the Index would therefore be ideally suited to a continuous monitoring of mobility patterns, but the actual *method* of recording and storing information is not suitable in its present form. The Index was substantially revised in 1962, and the nature of the changes makes it impossible to undertake retrospective analyses of previous movements. At present only part of the requisite information is stored in punched form, and the fact that it may be divided between a number of different cards, none of which can be conveniently linked with any other, means that the Index in its present form would not be suitable for monitoring future movements. However, certain modifications in the methods of recording information could enable the Index to be used for this purpose, and the possible computerisation of records in the future would greatly enhance the sophistication of the resulting analyses. There are, obviously, administrative and political barriers to be surmounted before the Index could be used in this way, but these ought not to be invoked as reasons preventing further consideration of its potential value.

The designated area allowance: some underlying assumptions

A second major area which might usefully be reviewed concerns the assumptions inherent in the method by which the allowance is administered. The first general assumption is that a list size of about 2,500 represents the maximum number of patients for whom a GP can provide reasonable care, and that this figure is equally valid in all parts of the country. Second, the scheme assumes that average list size is a reasonable indicator of workload. The reason for trying to attract more doctors into particular areas can only be that the existing workload is assumed to justify extra manpower, and since the mechanisms of intervention (described in Chapter 2) are activated only when a predetermined doctor/patient ratio is achieved it follows that list size must represent the official indicator of the point where the workload justifies more doctors. Third, there is the assumption that the medical practice area (as defined by the Medical Practices Committee) is the most appropriate unit on which to base the administration of the allowance.

There appears to have been very little attempt to validate these assumptions, even though they may not all be accepted by those responsible for administering the allowance. With respect to the first assumption listed above, an average doctor/patient ratio of 1 : 2,500 may have been a valid criterion of designation in 1952 (although even at that time there was little systematic justification of its choice), but the pace of technical and administrative development has been so rapid during the last two decades that its continuing validity is far from obvious. Nor is it obvious why the same criterion should be applied uniformly to all areas regardless of their size, population density, or demographic and epidemiological characteristics. There is considerable scope for increasing the flexibility of the system by having a variable criterion of designation which could incorporate a fairly wide range of available information about an area in addition to its list size. Some concessions might then be made to suit local variations from one area to another. Ultimately, however, the ideal solution may require the abandonment of list size as a major indicator and the substitution of more sophisticated measures of medical need and workload. That these measures have not so far been incorporated into the definition of a designated area is an indication of the difficulty involved in identifying, measuring and monitoring them throughout the country, but there is abundant evidence from the survey that the failure of GPs to accept the second assumption above has resulted in fairly widespread scepticism about the allowance. Doctors in non-designated areas pointed out, for example, that they were as hard-pressed as their colleagues in designated areas sometimes only a hundred yards down the road, or that their localities were just as deprived and unattractive as those which qualified for the payment – often more so. This is indeed true, and it helps little to point out to such doctors that what their areas lack, and what precludes them from receiving the allowance, is a high average list size. We return to this theme later.

The third assumption, that the medical practice area is the most appropriate unit on which to base the administration of the allowance, raises the subsidiary question as to whether eligibility for the allowance should be based on individual or practice list sizes rather than (as at present) the average list size for an area. It was shown in Chapter 10 that the range of list sizes *within* areas is sufficiently wide to ensure that a fairly large number of GPs with smallish lists receive the allowance, and conversely that quite a lot of doctors with more than 2,500 patients are automatically ineligible because their areas are not designated. If the criteria for payment were switched from areas to individual doctors, the number in receipt of the allowance might increase by as much as 200 per cent (depending upon the qualifications stipulated for eligibility). But it does not follow from this that eligibility should be determined by individual rather than area list sizes, for the purpose of the incentive is to attract doctors into areas with high average list sizes and *not* to encourage them to build up and maintain large lists. It would, for example, be difficult to justify payment of the allowance to a doctor with a personal list of 2,750 if all other doctors in the area had lists below 1,500. Such a payment would merely represent an individual bonus to that particular person, and would not in any sense constitute an incentive to other practitioners to move into the area. Conversely, in an area in which all the GPs had large list sizes an incoming practitioner might be denied the allowance (if it were to be paid on the basis of personal list size) while his individual list was building up to the designated level, and this too would be difficult to defend.

It seems clear that, if the incentive is to be based on list size, it ought to be the list size of the area rather than of practices or individual doctors.[5] The crucial question, however, is: what is to be defined as an appropriate area for this purpose? The question goes to the heart of the problem, for the payment of the allowance to all doctors in an area can only be justified if the area is reasonably homogeneous in terms of the need and demand for medical care and the provision of services. Many existing practice areas fail to meet this condition. Their boundaries have been determined more by historical accident than by rational planning, and when they were first adopted as administrative units by the Medical Practices Committee in 1948 there were no indications that they would later be used to regulate a component of remuneration. The task of the Committee in those days was to indicate broad geographical areas within which adequate doctor/patient ratios obtained, and the practice areas were entirely sufficient for this purpose. When the designated area allowance was introduced in 1966 the same areas were selected as the basis for determining eligibility, not because they were deemed to be the best possible units, but simply because they were the only existing areas below the level of executive councils in which list sizes were under continuous surveillance. The difficulties which this has created were understood with remarkable foresight by the Working Party on General Practice in 1964 which, anticipating the possibility of a separate financial inducement in under-doctored areas, commented that 'it would probably be necessary to base a scheme on areas other than those separately classified by the Medical Practices Committee'.[6]

The main problem concerns the size of the areas: some are much too large and others are much too small. Forty-nine county boroughs in England were single medical practice areas at 1 January 1970, which means that in many of the major cities and towns of the country the incentive of the allowance (where it is payable) applies to the entire city, whatever the local conditions. Most large towns contain some attractive areas with entirely adequate medical services and some which are relatively poor and depressed, where the medical care resources are overburdened. By determining eligibility for the allowance on the basis of the average list size for the town as a whole, GPs in the attractive parts may receive an extra £490 or £750 (if the whole town is designated), and conversely, those in the truly deprived neighbourhoods may fail to benefit from the allowance (if the average list for the whole town fails to reach the specified level). Such an area is clearly inappropriate as the unit of administration, for it fails to delineate self-contained medical care catchment areas. It would, for instance, matter little to either doctors or patients in a badly understaffed suburb of a town that other GPs elsewhere in the town had quite small lists. The problem is not helped by the determination of local pressure groups to maintain the status of a large town as a single practice area in order to preserve the allowance for as many GPs as possible. In such instances it is often inexpedient (though legally possible) for the Medical Practices Committee to over-ride local interests and to reclassify the town into smaller units.[7]

Difficulties may also occur in very small areas, although in practice these are less common than the problems of large areas. For example, a practice area with 5,000 patients and two principals would probably be classified as an open area. The introduction of a third principal would reduce the average list size to 1,666 and would change the classification to a restricted area. However, if one of the two principals retired, the average would rise to 5,000 and thus clearly justify the use of the designated classification. The pursuit of a consistent policy is difficult under such circumstances, especially in administering the allowance. Greater flexibility is available to the MPC in deciding whether or not to allow the admission of individual practitioners to restricted or intermediate areas (a restricted area, for example, may be reclassified as designated for one day only while a doctor is appointed with a type D initial practice allowance), but the same degree of discretion is apparently not exercised in determining area eligibility for the allowance. The long period of time during which an area must remain designated before the allowance is actually paid means that its incentive value is virtually eliminated in small areas where the addition or loss of one practitioner can alter the classification by one or more grades.

The designated areas: co-ordination in policy

We conclude this first part of the chapter by drawing attention to the fragmentation of responsibility over the development of policies for the designated areas. The above analysis indicates three inter-related elements which ought rationally to be considered in relation to each other in decisions affecting the designated areas. These elements are: the form which the incentives should take, the financial value which should be placed upon them, and the areas within which they should operate. In fact the responsibility for determining each of these elements is dispersed among different groups. The nature of the incentives is the outcome of negotiations between the British Medical Association and the Department of Health and Social Security; the value of the incentives is determined by the Review Body on Doctors' and Dentists' Remuneration (subject to final approval by the Government); and the areas within which they operate are fixed by the Medical Practices Committee. Moreover, the Review Body and the MPC constantly emphasise (probably quite rightly) their complete independence of both the BMA and the DHSS: neither is in any sense a sub-division of any government department. Interlinked with this fragmentation of responsibility is the system, described in Chapter 2, whereby executive councils and local medical committees collaborate with the Medical Practices Committee in deciding whether extra doctors are needed in any locality.

Many of the implications of this remarkable situation have been discussed at earlier points in the book. One which might appropriately be mentioned here concerns the difficulties of collecting and disseminating relevant data about manpower needs and use. Each of the groups involved in the process requires information, but there is no central information system to ensure that similar data are available to them. Consequently the way in which information is assembled, and the kind of information which each group considers to be relevant, lacks consistency and uniformity. It is, moreover, probable that communications between each group are insufficiently formal to ensure that information passed to, say, the Review Body through its secretariat in the Office of Manpower Economics, is also made available to the Medical Practices Committee. This weakness may be exacerbated when the reorganisation of the health service is made in 1974, for all the plans so far revealed propose that, in spite of the general emphasis on co-ordinated planning and the development of adequate information systems, the structure described above will remain virtually unchanged.[8] The Review Body and the MPC will continue to fulfil their existing tasks, the executive councils will be replaced by similar family practitioner committees, and equivalents of the local medical committees will be created. As more and more health service planning adopts an increasingly rational perspective the anomalies of this particular mode of decision-making may become increasingly apparent.

Influencing the spatial distribution of general practitioners: direct action

In this middle part of the chapter we concentrate on the more detailed aspects of the designated areas policy and in this section we examine the role of direct action. The term 'direct action' is used to denote the structure of incentives and controls that have been deliberately created to influence the spatial distribution of family doctors.

The designated area allowance

Apart from the difficulties associated with the philosophy and assumptions of the allowance, the main practical problem is obviously one of balance. Even the new levels of payment introduced in 1970 may prove to be too low radically to change the distribution of family doctors, but to raise them still higher would not only intensify the political and economic pressures surrounding the allowance, but would also bring them nearer to the point at which the disincentives currently operating in the scheme would render the allowance counter-productive. The Review Body has rightly been concerned that the allowance should not be so large as to cause inconvenience or financial embarrassment to doctors who might suddenly have it cut off, and the previous chapter has outlined certain other disincentives which are causing concern to many doctors. The evidence from our research suggests that the problem of disincentives requires more urgent attention than the question of levels of payment, and that if the former difficulty can be resolved then the current amounts payable may become more effective.

There are two major disincentives in the existing scheme, and these become greater as the value of the allowance rises. The first is the qualifying period of designation which an area must undergo before it attracts the allowance, and the second is the cessation of the allowance after the elapse of a concessionary period following de-designation. In the first situation the possibility of waiting up to three years for the payment after moving to an area, and even in some cases of not receiving the allowance at all, are substantial and obvious reasons why doctors may not be prepared to move. As the proportion of designated areas eligible for the allowance increases so this disincentive may diminish in importance, but it has been a significant barrier so far, and still remains one. It could be eliminated simply by removing the qualifying period and paying the allowance immediately to all existing practitioners in designated areas and to those who enter an area while it remains designated. As soon as the area is de-designated the allowance would cease to be payable *to incoming doctors*, although in order to overcome the second type of disincentive (discussed below) some basis must be established for continuing payment to those in receipt of the allowance at the time of de-designation. If the area was subsequently redesignated the allowance would again be payable immediately, either to all doctors in the area or only to those moving into it whilst it remained designated.

The machinery for monitoring continuous change in the existing classification of areas already exists, and as well as removing an awkward disincentive the elimination of a qualifying period would add sensitivity and flexibility to the manipulation of incentives and controls. To the extent that the allowance does function as an effective inducement it would be possible to concentrate the incentive immediately and directly upon areas which have difficulty in attracting manpower, and to remove it (for incoming doctors) when the requisite doctor/patient ratios have been achieved. The main objection in the past to suggestions that the qualifying period should be eliminated has been the alleged administrative complexity of coping with rapid changes in classification and of making the necessary adjustments to the remuneration of practitioners. Yet the abolition of the qualifying period would merely affect the number of doctors who *become* eligible for the payment, and not the number who *cease* to be eligible. If, as we argue later, some way should be found of continuing the payment for a longer period than at present, then the additional administrative burden would merely be that of noting the increased number of doctors who satisfy the appropriate conditions, and of adding the allowance to their remuneration.

The second disincentive in the existing scheme, arising from the cessation of the allowance after the elapse of a concessionary period following de-designation, is manifest in various ways. Doctors contemplating a move to a designated area may be deterred by the possibility of losing the allowance within three years of moving; those already in the area may be reluctant to admit newcomers when this would result in their loss of payment; and practitioners who suffer a loss of the allowance may have a substantially reduced desire to remain in the locality. It is obviously difficult to find any firm evidence that the disincentive really does work in this way because we do not know what would actually happen if it were removed. Nevertheless, the deliberations of the medical profession and the replies of the doctors in our surveys (some of which were reproduced in Chapter 12) point consistently towards the counter-productive tendency arising from this fairly abrupt cessation of payment.

There are various ways in which this second type of disincentive could be minimised. One solution would be to extend the concessionary period of payment beyond the existing period of three years to six or even twelve years. Another solution, proposed by the Health Departments in 1969, would be to continue the payment on a personal basis for as long as the doctor remained in the same practice or area, regardless of any subsequent changes in the classification of the area.[9] A third possibility would be to increase the financial incentive the longer the doctor remained in a designated area, by offering doctors moving into designated areas a loan to be repayed at an agreed rate, with a progressive reduction in the amount repayable for each completed year in the area.

Other financial incentives

As well as (or instead of) a simple addition to the basic practice allowance for doctors in specified areas, other items of remuneration might be loaded in order to maximise incentives. It has been suggested, for example, that each year spent in a designated area should count as one-and-a-half years towards superannuation,[10] or as two years towards a seniority allowance.[11] This latter suggestion is reasonably logical, since doctors in designated areas, having large lists, will presumably gain experience more rapidly than those elsewhere. Another way of distributing extra money would be through the establishment of differentials between designated and non-designated areas in the allowances available for the employment of ancillary staff. The principle is established in the reimbursement to GPs for the employment of assistants, and this particular differential (which at present amounts to £280 per annum) might be increased. The principle could be extended to other categories of staff, allowing designated doctors either to improve the staffing of their practices at no extra cost to themselves, or to continue with the same staff at a reduced personal cost. Similarly, a special locum allowance might be paid to enable the principal to take a holiday or study leave each year at no additional personal expense; or, more specifically, a sabbatical leave or research/study period might be allowed for each completed year in a designated area.

It is not difficult to think of different ways of distributing any extra money available for use as incentives. The ideas outlined above directly or indirectly put extra cash into the GP's pocket, either by enabling him to do more things for the same cost, or by increasing his income for the same workload. In principle, therefore, they do not differ substantially from the designated area allowance or loan scheme, and it is unlikely that their effect would be very different. If the value to the individual doctor is sufficiently high and if he is not deterred by any perceived disincentives, then it may matter little in which form the money actually reaches him. It is arguable that a form of endowment which directly enhances personal income (such as the designated area allowance or loan scheme) may be more attractive than one which either represents a deferred accretion of income (by providing favoured entitlement to superannuation benefits or seniority payments) or which is conditional upon the performance of certain prescribed actions (such as the employment of ancillary staff or the taking of study leave). In practice the distinction may not be sufficiently sharp to the individual doctor to constitute a differential incentive: if he is going to be substantially better off as a result of working in a particular locality, and if the prospect is an effective inducement for him, then it is perhaps of secondary importance in just what form the extra money is paid.

Non-financial incentives

The suggestions discussed above accept the principle and morality of cash incentives, but they raise the question of whether incentives should in fact be used to increase the personal wealth of GPs. A more effective, and certainly more equitable, policy might be to channel available resources towards the improvement of practice premises, equipment and staffing. Doctors would not be any better off personally, but they would enjoy larger practice subsidies, and would generally be able to provide a better service to their patients. The argument is not new. The Gillie Report in 1963 suggested the provision of premises in designated areas and of opportunities for hospital practice, public health work and medical administration.[12] The 1964 Working Party discussed the possibility of attachment schemes for health visitors and district nurses in under-doctored places, the provision of purpose-built practice premises, and the provision of adequate living accommodation for married junior hospital doctors in the hope of encouraging them to settle and to seek openings in general practice in such places.[13] More recently Townsend has suggested the introduction of a practice equipment allowance for the purchase of such expensive equipment as an ECG machine and vitalograph.[14] He also makes the suggestion that doctors who have spent a number of years in a designated area should be given preferential consideration when applying for more attractive posts. (In fact the MPC did urge executive councils as long ago as 1951 to give full consideration to doctors who, having spent much of their lives in substantial practices in heavy industrial areas, were seeking more modest vacancies in pleasanter areas towards the end of their careers.[15] Recent decisions by the Committee confirm that more than lip service is paid to the request,[16] but unless some kind of points system is introduced it is difficult to see how it can be fairly applied.)

The assumption which usually underlies such proposals is that designated areas are not only short of doctors, but also have poorer premises, equipment, facilities and practice conditions than places with better doctor/patient ratios. Since this is the case (the argument runs) it is logical that additional resources should be employed to compensate for these professional disadvantages. Some designated areas undoubtedly are comprehensively deprived in this way, but the results of our survey indicate that as a *general* proposition the assumption is dubious. The replies from the survey about practice conditions failed to differentiate consistently between doctors in designated and non-designated areas: in some respects the designated doctors were less favoured than their colleagues elsewhere, in others they were more favoured. Such findings invalidate the myth of widespread deprivation in the designated areas, but they do not necessarily cast doubt upon the potential effectiveness of non-financial inducements in levelling up the distribution of manpower. Doctors entering general practice will probably be increasingly attracted by the prospect of good practice facilities, and if the designated areas are that much better than the rest, so well and good. But it is desirable to maintain a balanced view of health care objectives, and the deliberate improvement of facilities in areas characterised by high average list sizes is not necessarily a sensible policy in itself. Not only would it widen still further many of the important gaps between designated and restricted areas (possibly leaving the latter as the new relatively deprived areas of the country), but it may also result in resources being used in areas which do not stand in the greatest need of them. We argue at the end of this chapter that it may be wiser as a long-term strategy to try to identify areas of medical deprivation as the units for special attention than to continue with the assumptions and objectives underlying the existing designated areas scheme.

Influencing the spatial distribution of general practitioners: indirect action

In addition to the various measures which may directly affect the distribution of family doctors, the results of the survey have highlighted further factors contributing to patterns of residential location which, if controlled, might afford less direct means of influence. But there is a dilemma, for some of the most powerful factors influencing the choice of residential location are those least amenable to deliberate manipulation, especially those associated with the connections which doctors have with particular areas (Chapter 7). Financial incentives may achieve some success among younger doctors if the correct balance can be found between effective levels and disincentive values; improved practice facilities may likewise attract younger men entering practice; but the location of a future doctor's birthplace, his home area, and his wife's family home are almost entirely beyond control.

There are, however, some possible pointers to policy choices in this matter.

The development of centres of under-graduate and post-graduate training in areas of chronic manpower shortage may be one way of harnessing the natural influence of existing contacts with an area on a doctor's choice of practice location. It is, obviously, impossible to control the areas of birth and upbringing of future GPs, and in any case it is impossible to predict on an individual basis which of today's schoolchildren will be tomorrow's doctors. What is open to manipulation, however, is the structure of opportunities which they have to develop their capacities, and the encouragement which they are given to choose medicine as a career. More energy might, for example, be expended on stimulating interest in a medical career among qualified sixth-formers in designated areas. Although there is no clear evidence of a relationship between the presence of a local medical school and the proportion of university candidates in the area who choose to study medicine, a local centre could undoubtedly contribute greatly to the effectiveness of 'recruitment' campaigns. Much of the initiative in meeting sixth-formers and in arranging a medical equivalent of the industrial short works' courses might come from the local medical community, supplemented where required by special campaigns mounted by central government and by local Youth Employment Officers.

Once the commitment to study medicine has been made by a school-leaver in a designated area, the offer of a place at a local medical school would reinforce the student's probability of remaining in his home area. The evidence for this was discussed at length in Chapter 7. It is the cumulative influence of community ties which led us in that chapter to reject the *principle* of the Todd Commission's argument about the irrelevance of settlement patterns to the siting of new medical schools and the expansion of existing ones, and although a great deal of detailed information would need to underlie any decision about the location of a new school, the results presented here are clearly relevant to the decision about establishing a medical school at Hull. On completing their basic training, prospective GPs might be exposed to propaganda about the geographical imbalance of doctors, and the social value might be stressed of young doctors spending the early part of their careers in the traditionally ill-staffed areas. The effectiveness of such exposure would naturally increase if the school itself were situated in such a locality. It would perhaps be over-stating the case to create the notion of 'VSO at home', but the idea of deliberately devoting a part of one's career to the cause of territorial equality in medical care might, if properly stimulated, appeal to the current egalitarian ethos of young professional people. Similar schemes are commonly run in developing countries, often with much success. They run the risk of encouraging a shifting and discontinuous service in the recipient areas, but in the context of the designated areas there may be compensating permanent gains of doctors who perhaps originally intended to practise for a short period only.

Medical deprivation and the planning of health services

This study has so far left untouched the question of whether the principles underlying the designated areas scheme are appropriate and realistic in the light of the known variability of needs and demands and the uneven distribution of services between communities of similar size. Our justification for the relatively narrow approach adopted in the study is that the research commission obliged us to examine current policies and practices, and thus to work largely within the framework of existing assumptions and objectives about manpower policy. We have, nevertheless, sometimes questioned these assumptions and objectives, and we conclude the book by drawing together some of these strands and carrying the discussion to a broader, and in some senses more fundamental, level.

General practice cannot function properly as an autonomous and self-sufficient medical care system: it complements and is interdependent with hospital and specialist medicine at one end of the socio-medical spectrum and with the public health and welfare services at the other. Recognition of this functional interdependence between different sections of the health and social services has been a major stimulus to the plans for the reorganisation of the National Health Service in 1974, even though the detailed proposals for change do not, at the time of writing, seem to integrate the general practitioner services wholly into the new unified NHS. But in principle it is logical that any proposals affecting the input to the general medical services should take account of the patterns of provision and functioning of other parts of the health and social service system, and of the effectiveness of the whole system in meeting the full range of medical needs in the community. It does not make good planning sense to develop criteria of adequacy and efficiency for one part of a system in relative isolation from the other interdependent parts of it. In practice of course it may be very difficult to avoid doing just this because of the complexity of the problems involved in attempting to do anything more ambitious.

The debate about the magnitude and distribution of the supply of GPs has paid little attention either to the total medical care needs of areas, or to the implications for other parts of the health services of policies concerned with the recruitment and dispersion of family doctors. In particular, the needs of areas for general medical services have been assessed mainly in terms of average list size, and considerable efforts have been made to attract family doctors into areas with high average lists and to discourage or even debar them from settling in areas with small lists. Yet it is already accepted that the size of the population of an area is not the only measure of its volume of need for primary medical care: qualitative features are acknowledged in the recognition that the elderly frequently require more of a doctor's time and should therefore attract a higher capitation fee (though this arises more in the context of providing a fair reward for doctors than as part of any explicit plan to encourage doctors to work in under-doctored areas). There are, in addition, many other demographic, geographical, social and epidemiological variables that are known to affect the demand for primary care; some of these have been discussed elsewhere in the book.[17] On the supply side, the structure and functioning of the full range of health and social services is likely to be as important as the simple number of GPs in determining how adequately the demand is met.

In a broad perspective, then, certain areas of the country are medically deprived in the sense that the existing services are unable to cope with the demands placed upon them, while others have a relative abundance of medical resources in relation to their needs. Hart suggests that there is an inverse association between the two: the availability of good medical care varies inversely with the need of the population served.[18] He writes: 'In areas with most sickness and death, general practitioners have more work, larger lists, less hospital support, and inherit more clinically ineffective traditions of consultation, than in the healthiest areas; and hospital doctors shoulder heavier case-loads with less staff and equipment, more obsolete buildings, and suffer recurrent crises in the availability of beds and replacement staff.' The exact magnitude of the association demands careful investigation, but sufficient data already exist to support Hart's basic thesis. The aim of a distribution policy in this situation should be to channel medical care resources into areas of medical deprivation in such a way that they catch up with the more favoured places, or at least to ensure that the gap between the favoured and deprived is narrowed. This is not always just a matter of getting more GPs: the additional financial expenditure involved in attracting more doctors to localities with large lists might be more efficiently deployed in certain circumstances in building up the stock of ancillary staff, improving practice facilities, adding to the number of home helps, health visitors or social workers, or expanding the range and capacity of the local authority social services.

The concept of a deprived area is well recognised in education, and programmes are currently under way to evaluate the infusion of substantial capital resources through the Educational Priority Areas scheme and the Urban Aid Programme into communities which not only have large classes in the primary schools, but are also deficient in the basic social support systems that children need in order to get the best out of their education, and which suffer from accumulated and multiple deprivations in housing, income maintenance, environmental amenities, economic opportunities and other social pathologies. It should be possible, in like manner, to identify areas of medical deprivation, which could then be singled out for equally comprehensive assistance in the health sphere. Such areas might well contain a large number of those which are currently classified as designated, but list size would be only one of the ingredients in the definition of medical deprivation. And just as the definition of a medically deprived area would transcend the narrow statistic of list size, so the desired remedy should go far beyond that of supplying one or two more GPs, which often does no more than to reveal further dimensions of need and deprivation. If the form of assistance given to these areas were to take account of the GPs' tasks and capacities within the total health services system it might then transpire that the real need is not always for more doctors, but sometimes for other workers and services which in the long run could do more to improve the overall standards of health.

These thoughts may seem wildly idealistic to the administrator trying to do something practical about an unsatisfactory situation with limited resources. He may legitimately ask who is to define the components used to assess medical deprivation? Who is to collect the necessary data and obtain and act upon indices of medical deprivation? What is to be taken as an appropriate area for the purposes of assessing medical deprivation? How much would it all cost? It would be useless to deny the practical difficulties of an approach of this kind, but it does serve as an ideal towards which we might strive. It is hard to accept the impossibility of going beyond crude population numbers in assessing the needs of an area for medical services, especially when considering the lengths to which the Inland Revenue, for instance, may go to arrive at an assessment of the tax due from an individual. It seems, moreover, that many of the practical difficulties may not be insuperable. The seeds of a monitoring system already exist in the Social Indicators movement, started in America and gaining ground in this country,[19] and the new General Household Survey initiated by the Office of Population Censuses and Surveys in 1970 also contains one section on health, sickness and the use of medical services. If the sample for this survey is eventually increased to an appropriate size and the validity and utility of the data can be firmly established, it might provide the basis for an information system far superior to anything that currently exists.[20] The point is that the necessary skills and techniques are available if the commitment is made to apply them to this end.

The question of finance raises a number of problems. The costs of collecting and processing the necessary data to monitor the working of the system would certainly be far greater than that spent at present on monitoring services. On the other hand, the same data could be of use to many bodies (such as local authorities) in their planning and monitoring activities, so that the costs need not all fall directly upon the health services. The costs of actually attacking relative medical deprivation may or may not be greater than that of working the designated areas scheme and other similar policies. The total amount spent on the health services is, after all, a government policy decision which takes into account many things other than the health and welfare of the country. The questions must be faced of how to distribute the current supply of resources in a more equitable way, and how far additional resources should be committed and distributed within the health services. The revelation of need via a sensitive monitoring system, even if it is primarily designed to effect an equitable distribution of whatever resources are available to the health services, may, however, have the effect of creating pressure for increased expenditure on the National Health Service, as has happened to some extent in education and recently in community care for the mentally disordered.

We have been discussing so far a total attack by the community on the problem of medical deprivation. This in turn is part of a wider problem of area deprivation. No progress, however, is likely to be made if we merely stand back and regard the problem in its complex and forbidding entirety. We need a strategy for learning. In practice this means breaking the total learning task down into manageable sub-tasks, so that we can move progressively nearer to understanding and manipulating the whole. This statement may seem to conflict with the opening remarks in this section, and indeed it does in a sense. There will always be some discrepancy between the ideal aim and the best possible practical attack on urgent problems. In approaching the sub-tasks, therefore, it is important to define the boundaries of the problem in a way that takes account, as far as is practicable, of the interdependence of these parts with the rest of the whole. It may be that by concentrating on the geographical distribution of general medical services (interpreting this to include not only the supply of doctors but supporting staff and facilities), and taking into account the sort of area features we have outlined, we will arrive at an understanding of the problem which is a definite improvement on the present situation, and which would not need completely rethinking when the task is widened, say, to include the provision of health and social services as a whole in relation to the needs of an area. We cannot of course be sure that this will be so because the system as a whole is not static in time – new inventions and ideas change the nature of the interdependencies between the various parts of the system. But that, in essence, has been the justification for this study.

Appendix A: the tables

Table A1 Distribution of unrestricted principals, and average list sizes, by type of practice area, 1952–70 (England and Wales)

Year	Percentage of principals in each area			Average list size in each area			
	De-signated	Open/Inter-mediate	Re-stricted	De-signated	Open/Inter-mediate	Re-stricted	Total
1952	44·0	49·2	6·8	2 851	2,184	1,581	2,436
1953	33·2	60·1	6·7	2,726	2,183	1,594	2,324
1954	22·8	69·5	7·7	2,741	2,228	1,546	2,293
1955	19·5	73·7	6·8	2,736	2,229	1,554	2,283
1956	18·2	74·7	7·1	2,711	2,234	1,548	2,272
1957	16·6	75·9	7·5	2,659	2,264	1,517	2,273
1958	15·7	77·1	7·2	2,627	2,247	1,594	2,267
1959	16·6	75·9	7·5	2,745	2,251	1,575	2,282
1960	16·8	75·5	7·7	2,723	2,257	1,603	2,287
1961	14·3	79·0	6·7	2,742	2,272	1,563	2,292
1962	14·7	76·7	8·6	2,744	2,297	1,608	2,304
1963	16·2	75·0	8·8	2,748	2,313	1,652	2,326
1964	17·9	70·7	11·4	2,768	2,359	1,747	2,362
1965	21·1	67·5	11·4	2,826	2,393	1,758	2,412
1966	25·6	63·4	11·0	2,845	2,407	1,807	2,453
1967	29·4	59·5	11·1	2,840	2,410	1,837	2,472
1968	33·3	56·5	10·2	2,819	2,395	1,811	2,477
1969	32·3	57·3	10·4	2,817	2,401	1,865	2,479
1970	31·8	56·7	11·5	2,791	2,391	1,884	2,460

Source: Annual Reports, Ministry of Health.

Table A2 The geographical distribution of principals in designated areas and the shortfall/surplus of principals, by standard regions and executive councils, at 1 October 1970 (England)

Standard region/ Executive council	Total number of principals	Principals in designated areas No.	%	Average no. of patients per principal	Shortfall (−) or surplus (+) of principals No.	Rate per 1m. patients
Northern region	1,315	750	57	2,528	− 15	− 4·5
Cumberland	99	—	—	2,200	+ 12	+ 55·1
Carlisle	32	32	100	2,571	− 1	− 12·2
Durham	296	211	71	2,735	− 28	− 34·6
Darlington	30	30	100	3,012	− 6	− 66·4
Gateshead	43	—	—	2,457	+ 1	+ 9·5
Hartlepool	31	31	100	3,175	− 8	− 81·3
South Shields	42	42	100	2,641	− 2	− 18·0
Sunderland	79	79	100	2,801	− 9	− 40·7
Northumberland	208	73	35	2,385	+ 10	+ 20·2
Newcastle-upon-Tyne	108	82	76	2,419	+ 4	+ 15·3
Tynemouth	23	23	100	2,672	− 2	− 32·5
Westmorland	40	—	—	1,771	+ 12	+169·4
Yorkshire N. Riding	137	10	7	2,082	+ 23	+ 80·6
Teesside	147	137	93	2,814	− 18	− 43·5
Yorkshire and Humberside region	1,919	950	50	2,549	− 38	− 7·8
Lincolnshire (Lindsey)	161	45	28	2,305	+ 13	+ 35·0
Grimsby	35	35	100	2,900	− 6	− 59·1
Yorkshire E. Riding	108	—	—	2,096	+ 17	+ 75·1
Kingston-upon-Hull	121	77	64	2,620	− 6	− 18·9
Yorkshire W. Riding	671	307	46	2,580	− 21	− 12·1
Barnsley	29	29	100	2,617	− 1	− 13·1
Bradford	121	56	46	2,636	− 7	− 21·9
Dewsbury	24	—	—	2,370	+ 1	+ 17·6
Doncaster	40	40	100	2,650	− 2	− 18·9
Halifax	35	35	100	2,638	− 2	− 21·7
Huddersfield	50	50	100	2,604	− 2	− 15·4
Leeds	200	73	37	2,576	− 6	− 11·6
Rotherham	30	30	100	2,895	− 5	− 57·6
Sheffield	205	147	72	2,681	− 15	− 27·3
Wakefield	27	26	96	2,631	− 1	− 14·1
York	62	—	—	2,283	+ 5	+ 35·3
East Midland region	1,351	596	44	2,596	− 52	− 14·8
Derbyshire	261	103	39	2,577	− 8	− 11·9
Derby	88	87	99	2,658	− 7	− 29·6
Leicestershire	188	68	36	2,555	− 4	− 8·3
Leicester	121	—	—	2,689	− 9	− 27·7
Lincolnshire (Holland)	41	22	54	2,493	—	—
Lincolnshire (Kesteven)	64	18	28	2,312	+ 5	+ 33·8
Lincoln	35	33	94	2,450	+ 1	+ 11·9

Table A2 continued

Standard region/ Executive council	Total number of principals	Principals in designated areas No.	%	Average no. of patients per principal	Shortfall (−) or surplus (+) of principals No.	Rate per 1m. patients
Northamptonshire	128	50	39	2,577	− 4	− 12·1
Northampton	57	—	—	2,547	− 1	− 6·9
Notts County and City	368	215	58	2,671	− 25	− 25·4
East Anglian region	702	118	17	2,336	+ 46	+ 28·0
Cambridgeshire	130	11	8	2,345	+ 8	+ 26·2
Huntingdonshire	73	28	38	2,544	− 1	− 5·4
Norfolk	183	—	—	2,244	+ 19	+ 46·3
Great Yarmouth	25	25	100	2,501	—	—
Norwich	57	—	—	2,300	+ 5	+ 38·1
Suffolk, East	110	—	—	2,142	+ 16	+ 67·9
Ipswich	54	54	100	2,628	− 3	− 21·1
Suffolk, West	70	—	—	2,393	+ 3	+ 17·9
South-Eastern region	7,441	1,452	20	2,427	+217	+ 12·0
Bedfordshire and Luton	178	18	10	2,734	− 17	− 34·9
Berkshire	206	53	26	2,436	+ 5	+ 10·0
Reading	67	—	—	2,456	+ 1	+ 6·1
Buckinghamshire	227	84	37	2,572	− 7	− 12·0
Essex	439	183	42	2,606	− 19	− 16·6
Southend-on-Sea	68	44	65	2,582	− 2	− 11·4
Hampshire	408	53	13	2,363	+ 22	+ 22·8
Bournemouth	77	—	—	2,088	+ 13	+ 80·9
Portsmouth	87	—	—	2,343	+ 5	+ 24·5
Southampton	94	—	—	2,567	− 3	− 12·4
Hertfordshire	371	168	45	2,643	− 21	− 21·4
Isle of Wight	50	—	—	2,122	+ 8	+ 75·4
London, Inner	1,437	—	—	2,295	+118	+ 35·8
London, North-East	470	266	57	2,543	− 8	− 6·7
London, SE. and Kent	772	342	44	2,544	− 14	− 7·1
London, SW. and Surrey	860	145	17	2,388	+ 38	+ 18·5
Middlesex	906	81	9	2,454	+ 16	+ 7·2
Oxford County and City	160	15	9	2,270	+ 15	+ 41·3
Sussex, East	199	—	—	2,168	+ 26	+ 60·3
Brighton	86	—	—	2,189	+ 11	+ 58·4
Eastbourne	31	—	—	2,189	+ 4	+ 59·0
Hastings	31	—	—	2,428	+ 1	+ 13·3
Sussex, West	217	—	—	2,241	+ 23	+ 47·3
South-Western region	1,723	140	8	2,241	+179	+ 46·4
Cornwall	181	—	—	2,089	+ 26	+ 67·1
Devon, Exeter, Torbay	317	—	—	2,038	+ 59	+ 91·3
Plymouth	106	—	—	2,323	+ 7	+ 28·4
Dorset	160	—	—	2,197	+ 19	+ 54·1
Gloucester County and City	281	24	9	2,292	+ 23	+ 35·7

Table A2 continued

Standard region/ Executive council	Total number of principals	Principals in designated areas No.	%	Average no. of patients per principal	Shortfall (−) or surplus (+) of principals No.	Rate per 1m. patients
Bristol	186	64	34	2,408	+ 7	+ 15·6
Isles of Scilly	2	—	—	1,026	+ 1	+487·6
Somerset	261	7	3	2,244	+ 27	+ 46·1
Bath	41	—	—	2,304	+ 3	+ 31·8
Wiltshire	188	45	24	2,477	+ 2	+ 4·3
West Midland region	2,004	1,332	66	2,608	− 87	− 16·6
Herefordshire	64	—	—	2,111	+ 10	+ 74·0
Salop	150	20	13	2,286	+ 13	+ 37·9
Staffordshire	248	163	66	2,682	− 18	− 27·1
Burton-on-Trent	24	24	100	2,758	− 2	− 30·2
Stoke-on-Trent	104	104	100	2,798	− 12	− 41·3
Walsall	67	67	100	2,980	− 13	− 65·1
Warley	74	73	99	2,506	—	—
West Bromwich	61	61	100	2,800	− 7	− 41·0
Wolverhampton	100	100	100	2,794	− 12	− 43·0
Warwickshire	269	149	55	2,603	− 11	− 15·7
Birmingham	443	325	73	2,579	− 14	− 12·3
Coventry	132	132	100	2,728	− 12	− 33·3
Worcestershire	174	20	11	2,406	+ 7	+ 16·7
Dudley	61	61	100	2,954	− 11	− 61·0
Worcester	33	33	100	2,709	− 3	− 33·6
North-Western region	2,644	1,101	42	2,578	− 83	− 12·2
Cheshire	417	114	27	2,484	+ 3	+ 2·9
Birkenhead	60	—	—	2,483	+ 1	+ 6·7
Chester	37	—	—	2,547	− 1	− 10·6
Stockport	62	62	100	2,512	—	—
Wallasey	45	—	—	2,360	+ 3	+ 28·3
Lancashire	853	509	60	2,698	− 67	− 29·1
Barrow-in-Furness	27	—	—	2,513	—	—
Blackburn	41	41	100	2,867	− 6	− 51·0
Blackpool	68	—	—	2,356	+ 4	+ 25·0
Bolton	62	62	100	2,831	− 8	− 45·6
Bootle	32	32	100	2,671	− 2	− 23·4
Burnley	38	—	—	2,319	+ 3	+ 34·0
Bury	25	25	100	2,883	− 4	− 55·5
Liverpool	279	1	—	2,465	+ 4	+ 5·8
Manchester	246	51	21	2,475	+ 3	+ 4·9
Oldham	48	48	100	2,736	− 5	− 38·1
Preston	52	50	96	2,557	− 1	− 7·5
Rochdale	32	32	100	2,939	− 6	− 63·8
St Helens	41	41	100	3,016	− 8	− 64·7
Salford	69	—	—	2,237	+ 7	+ 45·3
Southport	39	—	—	2,322	+ 3	+ 33·1
Warrington	38	—	—	2,576	− 1	− 10·2
Wigan	33	33	100	2,622	− 2	− 23·1
TOTAL, ENGLAND	19,099	6,439	34	2,478	+168	+ 3·6

Source: Annual Report and unpublished statistics, DHSS.

*Table A3 Response rates, by divisions**

Division	Total no. in division	Removed from sample	Sample denom-inator	Response rates: First mailing No.	First mailing % of total	Second mailing No.	Second mailing % of total	Second mailing % of remainder	Third mailing No.	Third mailing % of total	Third mailing % of remainder	Total No.	Total %
Western	442	32	410	274	66·8	61	14·9	44·9	17	4·1	22·7	352	85·9
East Midland	280	21	259	168	64·9	37	14·3	40·7	13	5·0	24·1	218	84·2
North-Eastern	311	18	293	196	66·9	51	17·4	52·6	15	5·1	32·6	262	89·4
Eastern	456	31	425	253	59·5	65	15·3	37·8	25	5·9	23·4	343	80·7
Southern	382	18	364	234	64·3	62	17·0	47·7	17	4·7	25·0	313	86·0
North-Western	295	15	280	174	61·9	35	12·5	33·0	24	8·6	33·8	233	83·2
TOTAL	2,166	135	2,031	1,299	64·0	311	15·3	42·5	111	5·5	26·4	1,721	84·7

* The Divisions referred to here are the DHSS Divisions within which the general medical services are administered. They do not correspond with any other geographical unit used in this study, and were used solely for reasons of administrative convenience.

Table A4 The proportions of doctors who responded, by type of area, sex, age, number of principals in the practice, and list size

	In designated areas		In non-designated areas	
	Number of doctors approached	Percentage who responded	Number of doctors approached	Percentage who responded
Classification of area				
Designated, + allowance	497	83·3	—	—
Designated, – allowance	319	85·6	—	—
Intermediate	—	—	304	84·5
Restricted	—	—	175	89·7
Open	—	—	736	84·2
Sex				
Male	764	85·2	1,097	85·4
Female	52	69·2	118	82·2
Age				
Below 30	7	100·0	12	91·7
30–34	58	91·4	89	88·8
35–39	126	91·3	128	87·5
40–44	166	84·9	224	90·2
45–49	139	82·7	210	87·6
50–54	125	85·6	173	85·5
55–59	87	78·2	175	82·9
60–64	57	82·5	100	80·0
65+	51	66·7	104	70·2
Principals in practice				
1	147	77·6	296	75·3
2	220	80·0	337	85·8
3	229	89·5	261	90·0
4	116	85·3	178	88·2
5	62	93·5	73	89·0
6 or more	42	83·3	70	92·9
List size				
Under 1,000	12	25·0	32	62·5
1,000–1,599	22	77·3	118	81·4
1,600–2,199	65	78·5	326	83·1
2,200–2,599	126	83·3	321	88·8
2,600–3,199	348	86·5	293	87·4
3,200–3,799	220	86·8	106	83·0
3,800+	23	82·6	19	94·7

Table A5 Number of different positions held in general practice and present age of doctors

Present age	Number of positions held in general practice 1	2	3+	Not known	Number of doctors (= 100%)	Mean number of positions
Designated sample	%	%	%	%		
Below 30	86	—	14	—	7	1·3
30–34	55	34	11	—	53	1·6
35–39	45	34	21	—	115	1·8
40–44	33	40	27	—	141	2·1
45–49	39	32	29	—	115	2·0
50–54	39	43	16	2	107	1·8
55–59	44	35	21	—	68	1·9
60+	39	31	30	—	81	2·1
All ages	41	36	23	—	687	1·9
Non-designated sample	%	%	%	%		
Below 30	82	18	—	—	11	1·2
30–34	49	41	10	—	79	1·6
35–39	43	31	26	—	112	2·0
40–44	38	30	32	—	202	2·1
45–49	42	33	25	—	184	1·9
50–54	41	36	22	1	148	1·9
55–59	46	30	24	—	145	1·9
60+	48	25	24	3	153	1·9
All ages	44	32	24	—	1,034	1·9

Table A6 Mobility type and present age of doctors

Mobility type	Present age: Designated sample under 40	Designated sample 40 and above	Non-designated sample under 40	Non-designated sample 40 and above
	%	%	%	%
No mobility	50	38	48	43
Mobility within county	15	16	15	15
Mobility within region	8	8	13	8
Mobility between regions	27	37	24	33
Not known	—	1	—	1
Number of doctors (= 100%)	175	512	202	832

Table A7 Present age and age at starting current position of all doctors who had changed practices at least once

Age at starting current position	Present age: Below 35	35–39	40–49	50–59	60+	All ages
Designated sample	%	%	%	%	%	%
Below 30	56	38	35	12	35	31
30–34	44	56	35	44	27	40
35–39	—	6	20	26	10	17
40–49	—	—	10	15	14	9
50+	—	—	—	3	12	3
Not known	—	—	—	—	2	—
Number of doctors (= 100%)	25	63	164	101	49	402
Non-designated sample	%	%	%	%	%	%
Below 30	79	19	22	14	21	23
30–34	21	67	43	36	24	40
35–39	—	14	24	26	17	21
40–49	—	—	11	16	20	12
50+	—	—	—	7	15	4
Not known	—	—	—	1	3	—
Number of doctors (= 100%)	42	64	231	165	75	577

Table A8 Losses, gains and net balance of internal migration; immigration; and total balance of movement, by standard regions (population estimates for England, 1968)

Standard region	(1) Doctors first practising in region	(2)	(3) Internal migration	(4)	(5)	(6)	(7)	(8)	(9) Immigrant doctors from abroad and unknown regions	(10)	(11) Doctors currently practising in region (1968)	(12)
			Losses		Gains		Net balance					
	No.	(=100%)	No.	%	No.	%	No.	%	No.	%	No.	%
North	1,250	100	293	23·4	234	18·7	− 59	− 4·7	130	10·4	1,321	105·7
Yorkshire/Humberside	1,757	100	537	30·5	343	19·5	−194	−11·1	127	7·2	1,690	96·3
East Midlands	1,187	100	421	35·4	613	51·6	+192	+16·2	122	10·3	1,501	126·4
East Anglia	624	100	170	27·2	201	32·2	+ 31	+ 5·0	35	5·6	690	110·6
South-East	6,495	100	999	15·4	1,247	19·2	+248	+ 3·8	558	8·6	7,301	112·4
South-West	1,871	100	727	38·8	416	22·2	−311	−16·6	139	7·4	1,699	90·9
West Midlands	1,940	100	632	32·6	502	25·9	−130	− 6·7	132	6·8	1,942	100·1
North-West	2,185	100	389	17·8	612	28·0	+223	+10·2	198	9·1	2,606	119·2
TOTAL, ENGLAND	17,309	100	4,168	24·1	4,168	24·1	0	0	1,441	8·3	18,750	108·3

Note All percentages are based on the number of doctors first practising in each region.

Table A9 *Net balance of internal movement between standard regions (population estimates for England, 1968)*

	North	Yorkshire/ Humberside	E. Midlands	E. Anglia	S. East	S. West	W. Midlands	N. West	Total
North		−2	−2	−2	−62	+23	−1	−13	−59
Yorkshire/ Humberside	+2		−9	+7	−41	−3	−22	−128	−194
East Midlands	+2	+9		+1	+79	+11	+93	−3	+192
East Anglia	+2	−7	−1		−9	+20	0	+26	+31
South-East	+62	+41	−79	+9		+211	+64	−60	+248
South-West	−23	+3	−11	−20	−211		−59	+10	−311
West Midlands	+1	+22	−93	0	−64	+59		−55	−130
North-West	+13	+128	+3	−26	+60	−10	+55		+223

Note The table is read across the rows. Thus, the Northern region shows a net oss of 2 doctors to Yorkshire/Humberside, the East Midlands and East Anglia, a net loss of 62 to the South-East, a net gain of 23 from the South-West, and so on.

Table A10 Standard region of first and current practices (population estimates for England, 1968)

Standard region of first practice	Standard region of current practice (1968)								Total
	North	Yorkshire/ Humberside	E. Midland	E. Anglia	SE.	SW.	W. Midland	NW.	
North	957	54	20	2	114	20	19	64	1,250
Yorkshire/Humberside	52	1,220	72	19	106	40	50	198	1,757
East Midlands	18	63	766	19	156	20	60	85	1,187
East Anglia	—	26	20	454	85	29	10	—	624
South-East	52	65	235	76	5,496	217	184	170	6,495
South-West	43	37	31	49	428	1,144	139	—	1,871
West Midlands	18	28	153	10	248	80	1,308	95	1,940
North-West	51	70	82	26	110	10	40	1,796	2,185
Outside England	113	117	112	33	480	119	132	184	1,290
Not known	17	10	10	2	78	20	—	14	151
TOTAL	1,321	1,690	1,501	690	7,301	1,699	1,942	2,606	18,750

Table A11 Adequacy of regions and counties on growth factors (see text, p. 72, for details)

Growth factor	Inadequate	Super-adequate
Capacity to attract new doctors	EAST MIDLANDS, NORTH-WEST, Durham, Derbyshire, Leicestershire, Northamptonshire, Huntingdonshire, Essex, Hertfordshire, SE. London/Kent, Worcestershire, Lancashire, Nottinghamshire	SOUTH-WEST, Northumberland, Hampshire, Inner London, SW. London/ Surrey, Cornwall, Dorset, Gloucestershire, Somerset, Shropshire, Norfolk
Capacity to attract mobile doctors	NORTH, YORKSHIRE/ HUMBERSIDE, West Riding of Yorkshire	EAST ANGLIA, Cumberland, Cornwall, Devonshire. Somerset Wiltshire
Capacity to attract immigrant doctors	Buckinghamshire	Cambridgeshire, Devonshire
Capacity to retain doctors	YORKSHIRE/HUMBERSIDE, EAST MIDLANDS, WEST MIDLANDS, Bedfordshire, Buckinghamshire, Essex, Hertfordshire, Leicestershire, Staffordshire, Warwickshire	Westmorland, Norfolk, Hampshire, Herefordshire

Standard regions are in capital letters.

Table A12 Influence of birthplace, home area and medical school on region of current practice (graduates of English universities, born and with family homes in England)

	Doctors currently practising in that region				
Events occurring in same region	Designated sample		Non-designated sample		Weighted total
	No.	%	No.	%	%
Birthplace only	4	10	4	7	8
Medical school only	20	26	42	28	27
Home area only	4	24	17	46	40
Birthplace and medical school	5	50	9	38	41
Birthplace and home area	25	35	66	47	44
Home area and medical school	19	54	29	59	57
Birthplace, home area and medical school	165	71	226	66	67

Note Percentages are based upon the total number of doctors in each separate category. For example, the first cell indicates that 10 per cent of designated doctors whose birthplace was in a different region than both home area and medical school were currently practising in their birth region.
The bottom cell in that column indicates that 71 per cent of designated doctors whose birthplace, home area and medical school were all in the same region were currently practising in that region.

Table A13 Relationship between family home and medical school, first appointment and current appointment, by regions (percentages based upon weighted aggregates of designated and non-designated samples)

Standard region of family home	Percentage of doctors attending medical school in the region	Percentage of doctors currently living in the region	Percentage of doctors taking first appointment in the region	Number of doctors (= 100%)
North	63	56	65	123
Yorkshire/ Humberside	68	57	61	133
East Midlands	—	39	32	59
East Anglia	3	63	55	35
South-East	88	65	64	416
South-West	27	59	60	77
West Midlands	60	57	56	86
North-West	60	55	47	174
TOTAL, ENGLAND	65	60	58	1,103

Table A14 Relationship between home area and area of current practice, by time of marriage, social class, father's occupation and present age (percentages based upon number of respondents with family homes in England)

	Relationship between home area and area of current practice						Number of doctors (= 100%)	
	Same county		Different county, same region		Different region			
	D*	N-D*	D	N-D	D	N-D	D	N-D
	%	%	%	%	%	%		
Time of marriage								
Before entering practice	35	32	19	23	46	45	287	491
Before present post	42	35	26	21	32	44	41	71
After present post	55	53	24	21	21	26	63	88
Other	54	50	23	20	23	30	22	40
Social class of father								
I	46	42	18	21	36	37	160	307
II	37	29	23	25	39	47	115	185
III	35	35	25	19	40	46	111	148
IV	50	50	13	—	37	50	8	6
V	—	48	—	52	100	—	2	27
Father's occupation								
Related to medicine	48	55	17	14	35	31	116	186
Unrelated to medicine	36	28	23	26	41	46	292	496
Present age								
Below 35	44	26	23	19	33	55	48	80
35–44	38	39	19	25	43	36	180	231
45–54	42	33	20	19	38	48	117	213
55–64	39	41	26	24	35	35	54	127
65+	29	39	21	26	50	35	14	39

* D = designated sample; N-D = non-designated sample.

Table A15 Type of practice area and social class of father

Social class of father	Type of practice area: Designated	Open	Intermediate	Restricted
	%	%	%	%
I	32	37	44	47
II	34	33	27	27
III non-manual	15	15	12	13
III manual	11	9	8	4
IV	2	1	1	3
V	1	—	—	—
Not known	5	5	8	6
Number of doctors (= 100%)	687	620	257	157

Table A16 Type of practice area and time of marriage

Time of marriage	Type of practice area: Designated	Open	Intermediate	Restricted
	%	%	%	%
Before starting general practice	66	63	67	73
After starting general practice but before present position	14	14	11	12
After starting present position	15	16	13	11
Not known	2	2	4	—
Never married	3	5	5	4
Number of doctors (= 100%)	687	620	257	157

Table A17 Type of practice area and age of children at starting current position (married respondents only)

Age of children at	Type of practice area			
starting current position	Designated	Open	Intermediate	Restricted
	%	%	%	%
No children	45	44	42	42
Eldest child under 11	49	50	52	49
Eldest child over 11	6	6	6	9
Number of doctors (= 100%)	649	574	235	150

Table A18 Primary qualifications and type of practice area

	Type of practice area			
Primary qualifications	Designated	Open	Intermediate	Restricted
	%	%	%	%
M.B., Ch.B. or equivalent *only*	66	62	58	56
Conjoint or equivalent *only*	18	19	18	19
M.B., Ch.B. *and* conjoint or equivalent	13	18	22	23
Others	3	1	2	2
Number of doctors (= 100%)	687	620	257	157

Table A19 Median years in general practice, median years in current position, and median age at starting current position

	Type of practice area			
	Designated	Open	Intermediate	Restricted
Median number of years in general practice	16·6	17·4	17·1	17·5
Median number of years in current position	14·8	15·5	14·8	14·5
Median age at starting current position	30·5	31·6	31·6	32·4

Table A20 Type of practice area and appointments held outside general practice

Appointments held outside general practice	Type of practice area Designated	Open	Intermediate	Restricted
	%	%	%	%
Hospital only	12	13	13	19
Non-hospital only	35	37	34	33
Hospital and non-hospital	9	13	15	14
None	44	36	38	34
Not known	—	1	—	—
Number of doctors (= 100%)	687	620	257	157

Table A21 Type of practice area and direct access to hospital beds

Direct access available to:	Type of practice area Designated	Open	Intermediate	Restricted
	%	%	%	%
Obstetric beds only	37	28	24	22
Other beds only	4	9	11	17
Obstetric and other beds	6	13	22	22
No beds at all	51	47	42	38
Not known	2	3	1	1
Number of doctors (= 100%)	687	620	257	157

Table A22 Type of practice area and rating of communications from hospitals when patients are discharged

Communications from hospitals	Type of practice area: Designated	Open	Intermediate	Restricted
	%	%	%	%
Very good	10	6	7	7
Good	51	56	55	53
Poor	32	30	26	30
Very poor	4	4	7	7
Not known	3	4	5	3
Number of doctors (= 100%)	687	620	257	157
Mean score	2·7	2·7	2·7	2·6

Note Mean scores are calculated as described in the text (p. 99), and exclude 'not known' responses.

Table A23 Type of practice area and rating of opportunities for post-graduate or refresher courses

Opportunities for courses	Type of practice area: Designated	Open	Intermediate	Restricted
	%	%	%	%
Very good	32	36	26	25
Good	48	44	49	44
Poor	15	14	16	20
Very poor	4	4	5	9
Not known	1	2	4	2
Number of doctors (= 100%)	687	620	257	157
Mean score	3·1	3·1	3·0	2·9

Note Mean scores are calculated as described in the text (p. 99), and exclude 'not known' responses.

Table A24 Type of practice area and frequency of contacts with teaching hospitals

Contacts with teaching hospitals	Type of practice area			
	Designated	Open	Intermediate	Restricted
	%	%	%	%
Frequent	13	16	18	13
Occasional	32	36	34	26
Rare	31	28	30	32
Non-existent	22	18	16	28
Not known	2	2	2	1
Number of doctors (= 100%)	687	620	257	157
Mean score	2·4	2·5	2·5	2·2

Note Mean scores are calculated as described in the text (p. 99), and exclude 'not known' responses.

Table A25 Type of practice area and frequency of contacts with post-graduate medical centres

Contacts with post-graduate medical centres	Type of practice area			
	Designated	Open	Intermediate	Restricted
	%	%	%	%
Frequent	49	44	37	38
Occasional	31	36	41	36
Rare	11	10	13	12
Non-existent	7	7	5	10
Not known	2	3	4	4
Number of doctors (= 100%)	687	620	257	157
Mean score	3·3	3·2	3·1	3·1

Note Mean scores are calculated as described in the text (p. 99), and exclude 'not known' responses.

Table A26 Type of practice area and list size

	Type of practice area			
List size	Designated	Open	Intermediate	Restricted
	%	%	%	%
Less than 1,600	3	7	11	30
1,600–2,199	7	18	32	48
2,200–2,599	15	28	32	17
2,600–3,199	44	33	19	3
3,200–3,799	28	12	5	—
3,800 or more	3	2	1	2
Number of doctors (= 100%)	687	620	257	157

Table A27 Type of practice area and number of principals in partnership

Number of principals	Type of practice area			
in partnership	Designated	Open	Intermediate	Restricted
	%	%	%	%
1	17	21	20	27
2	26	27	28	31
3	30	25	21	18
4	14	15	16	13
5 or more	13	12	15	11
Number of doctors (= 100%)	687	620	257	157

Table A28 Type of practice area and ancillary help in the practice

Ancillary help in practice	Type of practice area Designated	Open	Intermediate	Restricted
	%	%	%	%
No help at all	3	4	4	10
Secretary/receptionist only	23	26	20	20
Secretary/receptionist and nurse(s)	39	38	44	30
Secretary/receptionist, nurse(s) and other worker(s)	25	22	24	26
Other combinations	10	9	7	14
Not known	—	1	1	—
Number of doctors (= 100%)	687	620	257	157

Table A29 Type of practice area and number of nights on call per week

Number of nights on call per week	Type of practice area Designated	Open	Intermediate	Restricted
	%	%	%	%
Every night	7	8	12	26
5 or 6	9	13	13	18
3 or 4	29	33	37	34
Less than 3	53	44	37	22
Not known	2	2	1	—
Number of doctors (= 100%)	687	620	257	157

Table A30 Type of practice area and mean rating scores of educational provisions, cultural amenities, shopping facilities, recreational facilities and housing availability

	Type of practice area			
	Designated	Open	Intermediate	Restricted
Educational provisions	3·0	3·2	3·2	2·7
Cultural amenities	2·7	3·0	3·1	2·6
Shopping facilities	3·2	3·4	3·2	3·0
Recreational facilities	3·0	3·2	3·2	3·1
Housing availability	3·0	3·2	3·2	3·0

Note Mean scores are calculated as described in the text (p. 112).

Appendix B: the questionnaire

1. Which Medical School(s) did you attend?

2. What primary qualifications do you have? (Please tick)
   - M.B., Ch.B. or equivalent ☐
   - Conjoint or equivalent ☐
   - M.B., Ch.B. *and* Conjoint or equivalents ☐
   - Other ☐

3. What other qualifications do you have? Please include all higher degrees, diplomas, memberships, etc., and state the year in which they were obtained.

Qualification	Year

4. Please complete the following table for all positions you have ever held *in general practice*, except as a locum. Include your present position as the latest one, and specify the number of years you have spent in it so far. A change of position means a change of practice,

Position	Year of starting	Location (town and county)	Duration (number of years)
1			
2			
3			
4			
5			
6			

and *does not include promotions within a practice.* If any position has been split between two or more locations, please state the location in which the majority of your time was spent.

5. Since full registration, how many years have you spent altogether in *full-time* paid positions in:
   hospital work? ____ years ____ months
   military service? ____ years ____ months
   other medical appointments *apart from* general practice? ____ years ____ months

6. What other medical appointments do you *currently* hold outside the provision of general medical services?

Appointment	Type of appointment
1	
2	
3	
4	

7. Do you receive a group practice allowance? (Please tick)
   No ☐
   Yes ☐

8. What ancillary help, either full-time or part-time, do you have in or attached to the practice? (Please tick all that apply)
   No ancillary help ☐
   Secretary/receptionist ☐
   District Nurse ☐
   Health Visitor ☐
   Other SRN/SEN ☐
   Social Worker ☐
   Other ancillary help ☐

9. Do you feel that the ancillary help provided in your practice is: (Please tick)
   most adequate? ☐
   adequate? ☐
   inadequate? ☐
   most inadequate? ☐

10. Are your main or branch consulting rooms in a Local Authority Clinic or a Health Centre? (Please tick)

	No	*Yes*
Main consulting rooms	☐	☐
Branch consulting rooms	☐	☐

11. How many nights of the week are you on call, on the average, for cases other than obstetrics? (Please tick)
    - Every night ☐
    - 5 or 6 nights ☐
    - 3 or 4 nights ☐
    - 2 or fewer nights ☐

12. Do you have direct access to any NHS beds where you retain full responsibility for the treatment of your patients whilst in hospital? (Please tick all that apply)
    - No beds at all ☐
    - Obstetric ☐
    - Medical ☐
    - Surgical ☐
    - Geriatric ☐
    - Other ☐

13. Do you feel that the direct access which you have to NHS beds is: (Please tick)
    - most adequate? ☐
    - adequate? ☐
    - inadequate? ☐
    - most inadequate? ☐

14. To which of the following facilities do you have direct access (i.e. not through a consultant or casualty)? (Please tick all that apply)
    - Full size chest X-rays ☐
    - Bone and joint X-rays ☐
    - Bacteriological examination of urine ☐
    - Glucose tolerance tests ☐
    - None of these ☐

15. Do you feel that the direct access which you have to diagnostic facilities is: (Please tick)
    - most adequate? ☐
    - adequate? ☐
    - inadequate? ☐
    - most inadequate? ☐

16. *In general*, how would you describe: (Please tick)

	Very good	*Good*	*Poor*	*Very poor*
Arrangements for getting your elderly patients into hospital?	☐	☐	☐	☐
Communications from hospital when patients have been discharged?	☐	☐	☐	☐
Your opportunities for taking post-graduate or refresher courses?	☐	☐	☐	☐

	Fre-quent	*Occa-sional*	*Rare*	*Non-existent*
Your contacts with teaching hospitals?	☐	☐	☐	☐
Your contacts with post-graduate medical centres	☐	☐	☐	☐

17. Do you use the following equipment in your consulting room? (Please tick all that apply)

Height scale	☐
ESR tubes	☐
Microscope	☐
HB meter	☐
Sterile gloves	☐
Proctoscope	☐
ECG machine	☐
Wright Peak Flow meter	☐
Equipped emergency bag	☐

18. How far do you live from your main consulting room? (Please tick)

Main consulting room as part of residence	☐
Less than 2 miles	☐
2–5 miles	☐
6–10 miles	☐
More than 10 miles	☐

19. What influenced your choice of this area as the one in which to practise?

20. *In general,* how satisfactory is this area for the needs of *you and your family* in the following ways? (Please tick)

	Very satisfactory	*Satisfactory*	*Poor*	*Very poor*
Educational provisions	☐	☐	☐	☐
Cultural amenities	☐	☐	☐	☐
Shopping facilities	☐	☐	☐	☐
Recreational facilities	☐	☐	☐	☐
Availability of suitable housing	☐	☐	☐	☐

21. Are you thinking of moving in order to practise in another part of the country (or abroad) in the next two years? (Please tick)

No	☐
Yes	☐

22. What considerations would be important to *you* in choosing an area in which to practise if you were to move?

23. Do you have any comments on the principle or value of paying an additional allowance of £400 per annum to doctors practising in areas that have been continuously designated for at least three years?

24. Where were you born? (Please state town and county)

25. What is your marital status? (Please tick)

Never married	☐	Now go to question 27
Married	☐	Now go to question 26
Widowed	☐	
Divorced	☐	

26. (a) In what year did you get married?
 (b) Please list the ages of your children, if any.
 (c) Where was your wife's/husband's home for *most* of the time before her/his marriage? (Please state town and county)

27. Where was your home for *most* of the time before you went to University? (Please state town and county)

28. What type of secondary school did you go to? (Please tick)
 Grammar ☐
 Public ☐
 Other (specify) ☐

29. What was your father's occupation at the time you were born?

Thank you very much for your help. Please return this questionnaire to Mr J. R. Butler, Centre for Research in the Social Sciences, University of Kent, Canterbury, Kent.

Notes and references

Introduction

1 M. H. Cooper and A. J. Culyer, 'An economic assessment of some aspects of the operation of the National Health Service', *Health Services Financing* (Appendix A). A report commissioned in 1967 by the British Medical Association and carried out by an advisory panel under the chairmanship of Dr I. M. Jones.

2 *Report of the Committee on Local Authority and Allied Personal Social Services* (Seebohm Report), Cmnd 3703, HMSO, 1968.

3 R. O. Walker *et al.*, 'Dentistry in the United Kingdom: a survey of the present position and future trends', *British Dental Journal*, vol. 118 (1965), p. 511.

4 P. J. Cook and R. O. Walker, 'The geographical distribution of dental care in the U.K.', *British Dental Journal*, vol. 122 (1967), p. 441.

5 A. Maynard, 'Inequalities in psychiatric care in England and Wales', *Social Science and Medicine*, vol. 6 (1972), p. 221.

6 This perspective is associated particularly with R. M. Titmuss, 'The role of redistribution in social policy', in *Commitment to Welfare*, Allen & Unwin, 1968.

7 For an early provocative statement see B. Abel-Smith, 'Whose welfare state?', in *Conviction*, MacGibbon & Kee, 1958. For more recent evidence see R. Holman, *Socially Deprived Families in Britain*, Bedford Square Press, 1970; M. Rein, 'Social class and the utilisation of health services', *New Society*, 20 November 1969; A. H. Halsey, *Trends in British Society Since 1900*, Macmillan, 1972.

8 B. Davies, *Social Needs and Resources in Local Services*, Michael Joseph, 1968.

9 R. E. Pahl, 'Poverty and the urban system', in *Spatial Problems of the British Economy*, Cambridge University Press, 1971.

10 T. H. Marshall, *Sociology at the Crossroads*, Heinemann, 1963.

Chapter 1 The history of the designated areas

1 R. M. Titmuss, *Problems of Social Policy*, HMSO and Longmans, Green, 1950.

2 H. Eckstein, *The English Health Service*, Harvard University Press, 1958.

3 *Planning*, PEP Broadsheet No. 222, 30 June 1944.

4 J. and S. Jewkes, *The Genesis of the British National Health Service*, Blackwell, 1952.

5 Ibid., p. 14.
6 *A National Health Service*, Cmd 6502, HMSO, 1944.
7 Eckstein, op. cit., pp. 148, 153.
8 G. Forsyth, *Doctors and State Medicine*, Pitman, 1966.
9 A. J. Willcocks, *The Creation of the National Health Service*, Routledge & Kegan Paul, 1967.
10 R. Stevens, *Medical Practice in Modern England*, Yale University Press, 1966.
11 Ibid., p. 223.
12 See p. 23.
13 *Lancet*, vol. 2 (1951), p. 331.
14 *Report of the Committee on General Practice within the National Health Service* (Cohen Report), HMSO, 1954.
15 *Report of the Committee to consider the Future Numbers of Medical Practitioners and the Appropriate Intake of Medical Students* (Willinck Report), HMSO, 1957.
16 F. Lafitte and J. R. Squire, 'Second thoughts on the Willinck Report', *Lancet*, vol. 2 (1960), p. 538.
17 *Report of Royal Commission on Medical Education* (Todd Report), Cmnd 3569, HMSO, 1968, Appendix 9, Table 3.
18 Review Body on Doctors' and Dentists' Remuneration, *Ninth Report*, Cmnd 3600, HMSO, 1968.
19 S. L. Morrison, 'Medical manpower in the National Health Service', in *Problems and Progress in Medical Care*, third series, Oxford University Press, 1968.
20 *British Medical Journal*, supplement of 4 February 1961, p. 37.
21 *Report of the Sub-Committee on the Field of Work of the Family Doctor* (Gillie Report), HMSO, 1963.
22 *Commentaries of Working Party on General Practice*, HMSO, July 1964.
23 *British Medical Journal*, supplement of 27 June 1964, p. 262.
24 Ibid.
25 Ibid., supplement of 5 December 1964, p. 201.
26 Ibid., supplement of 8 March 1965, p. 89.
27 Ibid., supplement of 20 March 1965, p. 101.
28 Ibid., supplement of 5 June 1965, p. 241.
29 Ibid., supplement of 16 October 1965, p. 157.
30 Review Body on Doctors' and Dentists' Remuneration, *Seventh Report*, Cmnd 2992, HMSO, 1966.
31 *British Medical Journal*, supplement of 18 June 1966, p. 262.
32 Ibid., supplement of 21 January 1967, p. 22.
33 Ibid., supplement of 25 February 1967, p. 60.
34 Ibid., supplement of 15 July 1967, p. 39.
35 Ibid., supplement of 24 June 1967, p. 177.
36 British Medical Association, *Memorandum of Evidence to the Review Body on Doctors' and Dentists' Remuneration*, November 1967.
37 Review Body on Doctors' and Dentists' Remuneration, *Ninth Report*, Cmnd 3600, HMSO, 1968.
38 *British Medical Journal*, supplement of 29 June 1968, p. 234.

39 Ibid., supplement of 5 July 1969, p. 3.
40 British Medical Association, *Memorandum of Evidence to the Review Body on Doctors' and Dentists' Remuneration*, October 1969.
41 *Evidence by the Health Departments to the Review Body on Doctors' and Dentists' Remuneration*, DHSS, 1969 (unpublished).
42 Review Body on Doctors' and Dentists' Remuneration, *Twelfth Report*, Cmnd 4352, HMSO, 1970.
43 *British Medical Journal*, supplement of 13 June 1970, p. 616.
44 Ibid., supplement of 4 July 1970, p. 39.
45 Ibid., supplement of 12 September 1970, p. 87.
46 *Report of the Review Body on Doctors' and Dentists' Remuneration, 1971*, Cmnd 4825, HMSO, 1971.
47 *Report of the Review Body on Doctors' and Dentists' Remuneration, 1972*, Cmnd 5010, HMSO, 1972.

Chapter 2 Controls and incentives

1 All regulations, fees and allowances quoted in this chapter are correct at 1 April 1972.
2 Paragraph 8(4)(b) of the Terms of Service (Schedule I to SI 1210), 1966.
3 Personal communication from the Department of Health and Social Security.
4 *Twentieth Report of the Scottish Medical Practices Committee.* Reprinted in the British Medical Association *Memorandum of Evidence to the Review Body on Doctors' and Dentists' Remuneration*, October 1969, p. 28.
5 Although practice *areas* in England are classified almost entirely by list size, the Medical Practices Committee usually takes account of a wide range of qualitative factors in deciding whether or not to admit *individual* practitioners, thereby modifying to some extent the rigidity of the classification. (Personal communication from the secretary of the MPC.)
6 Department of Health and Social Security, *Annual Report 1971*, Cmnd 5019, HMSO, 1972.
7 Quoted in Review Body on Doctors' and Dentists' Remuneration, *Twelfth Report*, Cmnd 4352, HMSO, 1970, paragraph 151.
8 Department of Health and Social Security, *Annual Report 1968*, Cmnd 4100, HMSO, 1969.
9 Medical Practices Committee, Annual Report 1967–8 (unpublished).
10 Department of Health and Social Security, *General Medical Services, England and Wales, 1970* (unpublished tables).

Chapter 3 The distribution of principals

1 For convenience, the phrase 'designated doctors' is used throughout the book as a short way of referring to doctors in designated areas. It should be noted, however, that strictly speaking it is only the *area* that is designated, not the individual practitioner.

2 For the purposes of this section the whole of Derbyshire has been included in the East Midland region and Poole (Dorset) has been included in the South-Western region. Otherwise the regional boundaries correspond with those defined in the *Abstract of Regional Statistics No. 6*, HMSO, 1970, Appendix I.
3 A geographical county comprises the administrative county and all county boroughs within its boundary. In most cases each administrative county and county borough has its own corresponding executive council.

Chapter 4 A survey of general practitioners

1 A. Cartwright, *Patients and their Doctors*, Routledge & Kegan Paul, 1967.
2 J. M. Last, 'The regional distribution of general practitioners and consultants in the National Health Service', *British Medical Journal*, vol. 2 (1967), p. 796.
3 J. M. Last and E. Broadie, 'Further careers of young British doctors', *British Medical Journal*, vol. 4 (1970), p. 735.
4 R. G. S. Brown and C. Walker, 'The distribution of medical manpower', in *Problems and Progress in Medical Care*, fifth series, Oxford University Press, 1971.
5 R. G. S. Brown and C. Walker, 'Motivation and career satisfaction in general practice', unpublished paper, University of Hull, 1971.
6 J. M. Beshers, *Population Processes in Social Systems*, Free Press, 1967. D. V. Donnison, 'The movement of households in England', *Journal of the Royal Statistical Society*, Series A, vol. 124 (1961), p. 60.
7 L. A. Brown and J. C. Belcher, 'Residential mobility of physicians in Georgia', *Rural Sociology*, vol. 31 (1966), p. 439. L. Benham *et al.*, 'Migration, location and remuneration of medical personnel', *Review of Economics and Statistics*, vol. 50 (1968), p. 332.
8 By having the returns sent directly to the University the respondents could be assured that their completed questionnaires would not be seen by any staff in the divisional offices.
9 Cartwright (op. cit.) achieved a response of 76 per cent with a longer questionnaire than that used here; Last (1967, op. cit.) achieved 87 per cent with a much shorter list of questions; Mechanic obtained a reponse of 73 per cent in 1966.

Chapter 5 The mobility of general practitioners

1 Memorandum from the Medical Practices Committee, MPC 2/51, 13 June 1951.
2 R. G. S. Brown and C. Walker, 'Motivation and career satisfaction in general practice', unpublished paper, University of Hull, 1971.
3 All areas outside England were treated as one single standard region for the purposes of this analysis.

4 *Report of the Royal Commission on Medical Education* (Todd Report), Cmnd 3569, HMSO, 1968, Appendix 19.
5 Secondary qualifications are defined by the question: 'What other (i.e. non-primary) qualifications do you have? Please include all higher degrees, diplomas, memberships, etc.'

Chapter 6 An area analysis of mobility patterns

1 The standard regions are here defined in the same way as in Chapter 3 (reference 2), with the exception that the whole of Lincolnshire is included in the East Midland region.
2 The discrepancy between the 1968 and 1970 figures is unavoidable. It was desirable in Chapter 3 to present the most recent statistics available, but the sample was up-dated only to 1968.
3 The form of the question enables us to identify only those respondents who had previously been in general practice in another country. There is no way of isolating doctors who had come to England after pursuing other medical careers abroad, but the number is probably quite small.

Chapter 7 The importance of community ties

1 K. R. Hill, 'Medical manpower: the need for more medical schools', *Lancet*, vol. 2 (1964), p. 517.
2 *Report of the Sub-Committee on the Field of Work of the Family Doctor* (Gillie Report), HMSO, 1963, paragraph 121.
3 *Commentaries of Working Party on General Practice*, HMSO, July 1964.
4 *British Medical Journal*, supplement of 7 July 1962, p. 2.
5 J. M. Last, 'The regional distribution of general practitioners and consultants in the National Health Service', *British Medical Journal*, vol. 2 (1967), p. 796.
6 *Report of the Royal Commission on Medical Education* (Todd Report), Cmnd 3569, HMSO, 1968.
7 R. G. S. Brown and C. Walker, 'The distribution of medical manpower', in *Problems and Progress in Medical Care*, fifth series, Oxford University Press, 1971.
8 R. G. S. Brown and C. Walker, 'Motivation and career satisfaction in general practice', unpublished paper, University of Hull, 1971.
9 Todd Report.
10 For the purposes of this survey the pre-clinical students at Cambridge University were counted as medical students in East Anglia.

Chapter 8 The doctor as a person

1 Review Body on Doctors' and Dentists' Remuneration, *Twelfth Report*, Cmnd 4352, HMSO, 1970.
2 M. L. Newhouse, 'Surveying the women doctors', *Newsletter*, 8 March 1966.

3 J. E. Lawrie *et al.*, 'Working capacity of women doctors', *British Medical Journal*, vol. 1 (1966), p. 409.
4 D. V. Glass and J. R. Hall, 'Social mobility in Great Britain: a study of inter-generation changes in status', in *Social Mobility in Britain*, Routledge & Kegan Paul, 1966.
5 C. F. Schumacher, 'The 1960 medical school graduate: his biographical history', *Journal of Medical Education*, vol. 36 (1961), p. 398.
6 S. Adams, 'Trends in occupational origins of physicians', *American Sociological Review*, vol. 18 (1953), p. 404.
7 R. G. S. Brown and C. Walker, 'Motivation and career satisfaction in general practice', unpublished paper, University of Hull, 1971.
8 *Report of the Royal Commission on Medical Education* (Todd Report), Cmnd 3569, HMSO, 1968.
9 *Report of the Committee on Higher Education* (Robbins Report), Cmnd 2154, HMSO, 1963.
10 See, for example: J. W. B. Douglas, *The Home and the School*, MacGibbon & Kee, 1964.
11 N. Rogoff, *Recent Trends in Occupational Mobility*, Free Press, 1953.
12 R. G. S. Brown and C. Walker, op. cit.
13 Todd Report.
14 J. R. Butler, *Occupational Choice: a review of the literature*, Science Policy Studies No. 2, HMSO, 1968.
15 P. W. Musgrave, 'Towards a sociological theory of occupational choice', *Sociological Review*, vol. 16 (1967), p. 33.
16 O. Hall, 'The stages of a medical career', *American Journal of Sociology*, vol. 53 (1948), p. 327.
17 Areas which were designated at the time of the survey may not have been designated when the doctors originally went to them, and vice versa; but it is probable that the character of most areas, which may be more important than the administrative label, has not changed substantially over the period in question.

Chapter 9 The doctor as a professional

1 D. Cargill, 'Recruiting to general practice in England and Wales, 1961–1969', *Lancet*, vol. 2 (1969), p. 1295.
2 Department of Health and Social Security, *Reports on Health and Social Subjects, No. 2*, HMSO, 1972.
3 A. Cartwright, *Patients and their Doctors*, Routledge & Kegan Paul, 1967.
4 Ibid.

Chapter 10 The doctor and his practice

1 Department of Health and Social Security, *Annual Report, 1971*, Cmnd 5019, HMSO, 1972.
2 It is technically possible for a doctor practising in a non-designated area to receive all or part of the allowance if 60 per cent of his

patients reside in a designated area. The exact number of GPs receiving the allowance under these circumstances is not known, but is almost certainly quite small.

3 A group practice allowance is normally paid where the group consists of three or more principals, who may or may not be in partnership, but who must work in close association from a common surgery. The fact that a recipient of the allowance need not necessarily be in partnership accounts for the small number of single-handed doctors receiving the allowance.

4 A. Cartwright, *Patients and their Doctors*, Routledge & Kegan Paul, 1967.

Chapter 13 Under-doctored areas: an assessment of current policy

1 British Medical Association, *Memorandum of Evidence to the Review Body on Doctors' and Dentists' remuneration*, November 1967.

2 Office of Health Economics, *The Personal Health Services*, OHE Pamphlet 7, 1963.

3 *Present state and future needs of general practice*, Reports from General Practice XIII, Royal College of General Practitioners, 1970.

4 M. Clarke, 'Recent developments in general practice: changes in list size and the effect on the practitioner's workload', *Update Plus*, vol. 1 (1971), p. 337.

5 This principle does not conflict with the possibility, discussed later in the chapter, that once a doctor has actually qualified for an allowance he may continue to receive it on a personal basis regardless of subsequent changes in his or his area's list size.

6 *Commentaries of the Working Party on General Practice*, HMSO, July 1964.

7 There have been a few instances in recent years where the Committee has succeeded in dividing large county boroughs into smaller practice areas. At the same time the Committee has also been grouping very small areas together, with a resulting tendency towards greater homogeneity of areas with respect to population size.

8 *National Health Service Reorganisation: England*, Cmnd 5055, HMSO, 1972.

9 *British Medical Journal*, supplement of 5 July 1969, p. 3.

10 Suggested by, *inter alia*, a GP respondent in the survey.

11 E. Townsend, 'Problems of designated areas', *Medical World*, September 1969, p. 19.

12 *Report of the Sub-Committee on the Field of Work of the Family Doctor* (Gillie Report), HMSO, 1963.

13 *Commentaries of the Working Party on General Practice*, HMSO, July 1964.

14 E. Townsend, op. cit.

15 Memorandum from the Medical Practices Committee, MPC 2/51, 13 June 1951.

16 Personal communication from the Secretary of the Medical Practices Committee.

17 See also, for example, I. J. Fahs *et al.*, 'Indicators of need for health care personnel', *Medical Care*, vol. 9 (1971), p. 144.
18 J. T. Hart, 'The inverse care law', *Lancet*, vol. 1 (1971), p. 405.
19 A. Shonfield and S. Shaw (eds), *Social Indicators and Social Policy*, Heinemann Educational Books, 1972.
20 See, for example, C. A. Moser, 'Some general developments in social statistics', *Social Trends*, no. 1 (1970), p. 7.

Index